Praise for *Fit At Fifty and Beyond*

"Reading your book has been an inspiration to me. (As) Ms. Senior America I am honored to be a spokesperson for all seniors across the U.S.... (The) book speaks to all of us, young and old, as we age to take charge of our lives and keep on keeping on eating right and exercising to keep our bodies in good working order... Having a good attitude goes a long way and eating healthy. If we will just exercise by walking, stretching, lifting weights, and a few floor exercises it will keep us fit and then enjoy the recipes in your book, we will live well..."

—Olivia Haley, Ms. Senior America

"Are you fifty (the "old half-way point")? Or perhaps beyond? Or coming up on it? If so, this nifty little book by Michael Gloth—with mouth-watering recipes contributed by Master Chef Rudy Speckamp—should be on your near-term reading list. Dr. Gloth, a distinguished internist and geriatrician at Johns Hopkins, has assembled a concise, to the point, on the mark volume of information and advice to help you live your life at the peak of health and enjoyment from this day forward. Rarely does such advice hit home with so much that is practical, scientifically sound, and integrated into life as best lived: take care of your body, mind, and spirit, exercise all each day with vigor and insight, eat well, and enjoy it all to the very end. So read on and live!"

—William R. Hazzard, MD;
Director Geriatrics & Extended Care,
University of Washington

"A gem of a book—inspiring, motivating, sensible, and filled with explanations about exercise, weight loss, and nutrition. Alternatives are offered to suit the individual as well as suggestions for getting back on track after detouring from the goal. The book reads easily, offers recipes, and has the feel of a good friend giving supportive advice."

—Brenda Kurz, Fitness Instructor

"This is a valuable contribution and will help those who read it... No matter your age or health status some form of exercise can help. Dr. Gloth's book provides practical and reasoned advice as how best to get started and sustain an effective program... easy to read and the sidebar notations are very useful and allow one easily to refresh what they read previously. I liked the recipes dispersed throughout the book as a reminder that staying fit after fifty is a well planned and sustained program of health behaviors, diet and exercise. Well done."

—*John Burton, MD, Director,*
Johns Hopkins Geriatric Education Center

"... flawless... a wonderful senior wellness health guide designed for the full body... uses real seniors to show its exercise and lifestyle photos... focuses on total wellbeing... a guide that is simple to follow and a lifestyle that could be followed well into the senior years. Each chapter ends with a summary of basic points and ideas expressed in the section... The exercises are simple and basic, and use only a few props (such as barbells and dumb-bells)."

—*Tina Samuels, Suite101.com*

"... enjoyable to read and extremely informative. Dr. Gloth makes a compelling case for why this age group must follow a sensible diet and include some form of regular exercise, but what I liked best about his suggestions was that they would result in changing my lifestyle without having to change much *about* my lifestyle to do it... Dr. Gloth's solutions are simple, tailored specifically to my age group, and motivating. The exercises are well demonstrated in photos and the low-calorie recipes throughout sound delicious. I can't wait to start!"

—*Linda Altoonian, author of* Living Agelessly

"This is a practical, enjoyable book on how to lose weight by combining diet and exercise. My wife and I prepared several of the recipes. I couldn't believe that they were actually healthy! We are going through every single one of these recipes and finding that each is better than the last. What is also unique about this book is that Dr. Michael Gloth describes, with illustrations, the kind of exercise that can be safely and effectively performed by senor citizens such as I... Read this book—you'll love it!"

—*Isadore Rosenfeld, MD,*
Professor of Clinical Medicine (Cardiology),
Weill Medical College

Fit At Fifty and Beyond

A Balanced Exercise and Nutrition Program

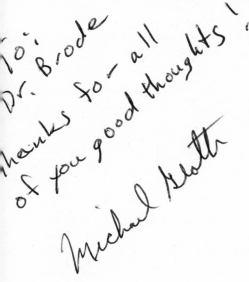

Michael Gloth, MD

with

Rudy Speckamp, CMC

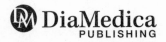

DiaMedica
PUBLISHING

DIAMEDICA PUBLISHING, 150 EAST 61ST STREET, NEW YORK, NY 10065
Visit our website at *www.diamedicapub.com*

Library of Congress Cataloging-in-Publication Data

Gloth, Michael, 1956–
Fit at fifty and beyond : a balanced exercise and nutrition program /
Michael Gloth with Rudy Speckamp.
    p. cm.
 Includes index.
 ISBN 978-0-9793564-7-6 (alk. paper)
1. Middle-aged persons—Health and hygiene. 2. Middle-aged persons—Nutrition. 3. Physical fitness for middle-aged persons. I. Speckamp, Rudy, 1946–
II. Title.
 RA777.5.G56 2009
 613'.0434—dc22

                                                                    2009010559

NOTE TO READERS
This book is not a substitute for medical advice and assistance. The judgment of individual physicians and other medical specialists who know you and who manage the treatment of any medical issues you may have is essential. Before beginning any exercise program, the advice of a physical therapist or qualified trainer is recommended.

Editor: Jessica Bryan
Designed and typeset by: TypeWriting

Dedication

This book is dedicated to my parents, Fred and Mary Jane Gloth, who are living testimony of the principles in this book, having remained active and healthy into their 80s. Fortunately for my five siblings and me, their example instilled these principles in us at a very early age!

Because I could never write a book like this without the support of my family, I also dedicate this to my loving wife, Maybian, and my children, Anna, Mary-Kate, Jane, and Molly.

Contents

Preface

Probably as many books have been written about diet and exercise as pounds have been lost and then gained back by people seeking permanent weight loss. Why would anyone consider writing yet one more book? The fact is that despite all the trees turned into paper to print books on health, and the many excellent books on this topic, a huge void remains in the information available for those of us who are over 50, even though we have very different nutritional and exercise needs in contrast to younger folks. *Fit At Fifty and Beyond* was written specifically to fill this void. It combines the knowledge of an expert in aging and nutrition with the skill of a master chef, and provides simple nutritional guidelines and healthy recipes that are specifically designed for those of us over 50. It will help you make food choices that are nutritionally balanced and delicious, without needing to calculate the amount of total fat or carbohydrates in each morsel you eat.

Metabolism changes as we age, and weight and exercise issues must be addressed differently. Many people reach 50 (and beyond) and wonder "What happened?" Without changing their eating habits, they have "suddenly" found themselves overweight and physically unable to do things that seemed easy just a few years before. For most people, the natural changes associated with aging—including a less active lifestyle— have led to increased weight and loss of physical conditioning.

When I was in college, I played softball and rugby, ran and worked out twice a day, and spent 4 years on the varsity wrestling team. At one point, I calculated that I was burning about 6,000 calories a day! After graduation, I stayed fairly active, but not at the level that I had during my peak in college. The decrease in activity and the age-related changes in my metabolism would have quickly translated into a huge weight gain, if I had not adjusted my eating patterns dramatically.

This book applies the principles that I've learned and followed myself. It provides basic information about how to avoid some of the effects that age can have on weight, and it also provides a basic "game plan" for getting into shape. For younger adults, it will serve as a preventive guide, so that the undesirable effects of aging can be avoided. For everyone, it provides hope for successful aging in an intelligent and sensible way.

In *Fit At Fifty and Beyond*, Chef Speckamp and I have combined our expertise in aging, nutrition, exercise, and cooking to provide practical suggestions for people 50 and older. Our recommendations for various exercise techniques and delectable recipes can be used as the basis for developing a successful plan for a healthy life. Chef Speckamp's sample recipes are proof that a healthy diet can be a mouth-watering experience, pleasing to even the most discerning palate, and will help you make nutritionally sound choices from cookbooks and restaurant menus. In addition to the recipes given throughout the book, the Resource section lists numerous cookbooks that can be helpful in preparing tasty, healthy dishes.

The chapters that follow will help you to look and feel better as the years go by—without sacrificing the pleasures of eating. *Dum vivimus, vivamus!* —"While we live, let us live!"

Michael Gloth, MD
Rudy Speckamp, CMC

Acknowledgments

First and foremost, I acknowledge Dr. Diana M. Schneider, my publisher, who worked so hard to make this book palatable to the general public.

Richard Lansing deserves some mention for recognizing the potential in the concept of the book and for referring me to Diana.

I acknowledge the tremendous help from my favorite photographer, Anna Gloth, who took the bulk of the exercise photos for *Fit At Fifty and Beyond*, and to Mary Jane Gloth and Fred Gloth, who posed for most of the exercise photos. Further thanks go to Mary Jane Gloth and Sherry Buchman for their review of the manuscript.

Acknowledgment is also due to Olivia Haley (Ms. Senior America 2008) who graciously demonstrated some of the exercises for the book and to Jonathan Norris (Electravision) who directed Ms. Haley's photo shoot and his assistant, Jacob Howe. Also, we are grateful to Williamson County Parks and Recreation Department, Williamson County, Tennessee, for providing facilities for Ms. Haley's photo shoot.

Finally, a warm thanks to my marvelous family for their loving support during the entire process.

About the Authors

F. Michael Gloth, III, MD

Dr. Gloth is an Associate Professor of Medicine and the Director of Outpatient Services in the Division of Geriatric Medicine and Gerontology at The Johns Hopkins University School of Medicine in Baltimore, Maryland. He has served on the National Advisory Council on Aging to the National Institutes of Health and on the Advisory Committee for the White House Conference on Aging. He has published numerous scientific publications on nutrition, represented the American College of Physicians in the development of the National Osteoporosis Foundation's Guidelines for Osteoporosis, and edited the *Handbook of Pain Relief in Older Adults.*

Dr. Gloth is an internationally recognized author and speaker, who has appeared frequently on radio and television and been quoted in such publications as the *Wall Street Journal* and the *Washington Post.* He has received numerous awards for his work in geriatrics, including the American Geriatrics Society's national Clinician of the Year Award in 2006.

Rudolph Speckamp, CMC

Rudolph Speckamp was trained as a master chef in his native Germany. He was a member of the U.S. Culinary Olympic Team and a member of the gold medal-winning 1998 team that competed at the World Cup in Luxembourg. His culinary accomplishments have won him 26 national and international gold medals, and he was named "Chef of the Year" for 6 consecutive years by *Baltimore Magazine.* Chef Speckamp is an American Culinary Federation Judge and serves as a Guest Instructor at the Culinary Institute of America.

As co-owner of Rudy's 2900, Chef Speckamp has earned further acclaim, including repeated DIRONA Awards, the Star Diamond Award from the American Academy of Hospitality Sciences, and the Certificate of Culinary Excellence from the American Culinary Federation.

Survival of the Fittest

AGING AND EVOLUTION

If you've had trouble maintaining your svelte figure of yesteryear, take heart. You're not alone. Terms such as "obesity epidemic" have surfaced to describe a large-scale (pardon the pun!) change in the people of many developed countries. The Centers for Disease Control and Prevention (CDC) website (http://www.cdc.gov/nccdphp/dnpa/obesity/trend/maps/index.htm) indicates that during the period from 1991 to 2004, obesity levels increased from no state having more than 20 percent of its population classified as obese, to levels that reached or exceeded 20 percent in 33 states. In 2004, a report in the *Journal of the American Geriatrics Society* reported that about three in eight people 60 years old or older in the United States would be obese by the year 2010, and that only about one in four would actually be in the normal range.

This tendency toward increasing weight gain has been in progress for centuries, as the forces of evolution have helped humans develop a natural tendency to store fat. Fortunately for us, over time, we have developed a higher intelligence that allows us to adapt. By recognizing the changes and adjusting our lifestyle to accommodate them, we can successfully maintain our well-being—and look good doing it!

> *The forces of evolution have helped humans develop a natural tendency to store fat.*

EVOLUTION OF SURVIVAL—"FITTEST OR FATTEST"

Except for the past century, our ancestors spent thousands of years in environments in which food was relatively scarce. As a result, we developed a natural tendency to enjoy eating, use energy efficiently, and store reserves in the form of muscle or fat, as if in anticipation of the next famine period. Historically, humans who were able to do this were more likely to survive, particularly during times when food was scarce. People who created fat easily were also more likely to survive and have offspring. In turn, their children had an increased chance of inheriting the tendency to eat more and convert their food into fat.

In times of famine, and even now during times of dietary restraint, an increase often occurs in cortisol levels and other biomarkers of stress. An increase in cortisol (an endogenous steroid) is also linked to weight gain when food is available.

It is easy to understand that the ability to store energy as fat has been helpful throughout history, since getting food was often a major challenge prior to refrigeration and mass transportation. However, relatively recent changes in farming, food storage, and transportation have revolutionized access to food and all but eliminated the age-old phenomenon of "lean years" for the majority of people in developed countries. Many developing countries are experiencing this food-availability phenomenon as well.

Compared to hundreds of thousands of years of evolution, the changes in the last 50 to 100 years have occurred in a Darwinian blink of an eye! Our bodies, which gradually developed into relatively efficient vessels for storing energy over thousands of years, are unable to adjust quickly by traditional means to the availability of food provided by modern technology. As a result, the relative abundance of food and the changes in access to food over the past century have led to our current problem of obesity.

If we use history as a prologue to the future, you might think that increases in weight would cause earlier deaths and that—from the standpoint of evolution and survival of the fittest—the trend toward weight gain would gradually reverse itself. However, this assumption is incorrect for two reasons. First, death related to obesity occurs late enough in life that it has no effect on childbearing and the transmission to our offspring of the tendency to store fat, so Nature will not correct this problem for future generations.

Second, we are able to adapt to this situation by adjusting our technology and lifestyle—as is true for many changes in environment and climate. In other words, we have the ability to change and thus avoid premature mortality. Fortunately, understanding what happens to our metabolism over the course of our lives can help improve our ability to stay fit and offset what is often described as the "ravages of time," which might be more appropriately considered the ravages of "repast"!

THE DEFINITION OF OBESITY AND THE PRINCIPLES TO OVERCOME IT

It is important to define what we mean by being "fit" as we grow older. Each of us must establish personal goals related to our outlook on life, quality of life, and personal desires. Some of us simply want to look trim and fit. Others might have the additional goal of increasing physical conditioning or strength. Whether you are trying to have "six-pack abs" or lose a few dress sizes, this book will help you reach your goal.

Let's first define what we mean by *obesity*. Traditionally, nutritionists define obesity simply as excessive weight ("body mass"), with too much of the weight consisting of fat. The *body mass index* (BMI) is a formula based on height and weight. It is equal to your weight (or mass) as measured in kilograms (one kilogram equals about 2.2 pounds), divided by your height (in meters) squared. As a formula, BMI = weight (kg) ÷ height (m)^2.

For example, the BMI of someone who is 68.2 kg (weighs about 150 lbs) and is 1.65 m (about 5'6") tall would be a bit less than 25.

Rather than spend time on calculations, simply refer to Table 1.1 on page 5 and line up your height and weight to get your BMI score.

A person with a BMI score greater than 25 is considered overweight by the U.S. Department of Health and Human Services, and above 30 is considered obese.

Before you get overly concerned about adding pounds as you get older, it is important to realize that *some* weight gain might actually be a *good* thing. There appears to be an association between survival and BMI. Data from the Baltimore Longitudinal Study on Aging showed that people with a very low BMI might have the same risk of death as those who have a very high BMI. The best survival rates are seen in people who have *slight* increases in weight as they get older.

A person with a BMI score greater than 25 is considered overweight by the U.S. Department of Health and Human Services, and above 30 is considered obese.

A tendency to lose some muscle and strength, and to add to the percentage of body fat—often described as increasing *body fat composition*—is a normal part of the aging process. Typically, exercise capacity declines as we age. The good news is that many of these undesirable changes can be minimized or reversed with proper diet and exercise, and it is possible to maintain or even increase muscle mass and strength as we age.

Slight gains in BMI might be a good thing, but ideally these gains should reflect gains in muscle rather than fat. Both men and women can increase muscle and reduce fat to produce this change in BMI scores.

The best survival rates are seen in people who have slight increases in weight as they get older.

If you want to age successfully, with improved strength and endurance, you need to understand the other changes associated with aging. Your body burns calories even when you are resting, and this process becomes more efficient as you age. In other words, the amount of energy your body uses at rest *decreases* as you get older.

TABLE 1.1 CALCULATE YOUR BODY MASS INDEX (BMI)

BMI	19	20	21	22	23	24	25	26	27	28	29	30	31	32	33	34	35
Height (inches)								Body Weight (pounds)									
58	91	96	100	105	110	115	119	124	129	134	138	143	148	153	158	162	167
59	94	99	104	109	114	119	124	128	133	138	143	148	153	158	163	168	173
60	97	102	107	112	118	123	128	133	138	143	148	153	158	163	168	174	179
61	100	106	111	116	122	127	132	137	143	148	153	158	164	169	174	180	185
62	104	109	115	120	126	131	136	142	147	153	158	164	169	175	180	186	191
63	107	113	118	124	130	135	141	146	152	158	163	169	175	180	186	191	197
64	110	116	122	128	134	140	145	151	157	163	169	174	180	186	192	197	204
65	114	120	126	132	138	144	150	156	162	168	174	180	186	192	198	204	210
66	118	124	130	136	142	148	155	161	167	173	179	186	192	198	204	210	216
67	121	127	134	140	146	153	159	166	172	178	185	191	198	204	211	217	223
68	125	131	138	144	151	158	164	171	177	184	190	197	203	210	216	223	230
69	128	135	142	149	155	162	169	176	182	189	196	203	209	216	223	230	236
70	132	139	146	153	160	167	174	181	188	195	202	209	216	222	229	236	243
71	136	143	150	157	165	172	179	186	193	200	208	215	222	229	236	243	250
72	140	147	154	162	169	177	184	191	199	206	213	221	228	235	242	250	258
73	144	151	159	166	174	182	189	197	204	212	219	227	235	242	250	257	265
74	148	155	163	171	179	186	194	202	210	218	225	233	241	249	256	264	272
75	152	160	168	176	184	192	200	208	216	224	232	240	248	256	264	272	279
76	156	164	172	180	189	197	205	213	221	230	238	246	254	263	271	279	287

The amount of energy your body uses at rest decreases as you get older.

This was helpful to our ancestors because age-related changes, such as being unable to run as fast, made getting food more difficult. Using fewer calories as they got older improved their chances for survival. Of course, for them, age 40 was relatively old! Consequently, especially for males, they would still be contributing to the nutrition, protection, and procreation of their social group.

If you continue to eat the same type and amounts of food as you get older, without increasing your level of activity, you *will* gain weight—and you *will* gain it mainly as fat. To counter this normal change associated with aging, you must reduce the number of calories you take in, increase the amount of energy you expend, or combine the two. As you will see, this does *not* simply mean eating less and exercising more.

If you continue to eat the same type and amounts of food as you get older, without increasing your level of activity, you will *gain weight—and you* will gain it *mainly as fat.*

Understanding some of the changes associated with aging will allow you to reach your ideal body weight with relatively little change in the amount you eat or the total amount of exercise or activity you do. By learning about the changes that occur as you grow older, you'll find it easier to improve your health, well-being, and general overall appearance. The information in this book outlines a process that is easy and involves minimal sacrifice. The advantage that this knowledge can give you will almost make you feel like you are cheating!

ENERGY EXPENDITURE AND LONGEVITY: NOT ALL CALORIES ARE EQUAL

Although the number of calories in the food you eat is important, you also need to recognize that the body burns calories during the process of digesting food, and some foods require far more effort to digest than others. This means that some foods with a greater number of calories might not be nearly as likely to turn into fat as others that actually have fewer calories. Knowing which types of food require more energy during the digestive process can make losing weight much easier.

Understanding some of the changes associated with aging will allow you to reach your ideal body weight with relatively little change in the amount you eat or the total amount of exercise or activity you do.

For example, a major source of energy comes from carbohydrates, which are essentially sugars. The simplest sugars include glucose and fructose, which are present in most fruit juices. These simple sugars can be chemically joined like links in a chain to form more complex sugars (Figure 1.1). They are called *complex carbohydrates*.

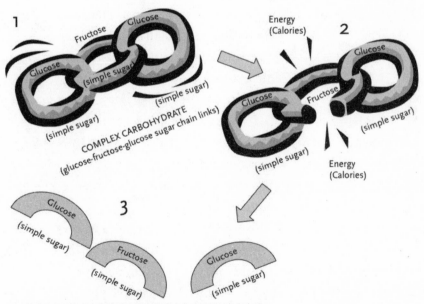

Simple sugars available for instant energy or conversion to fat

FIGURE 1.1 Burning calories to convert complex sugars (carbohydrates) into simple sugars. The body uses simple carbohydrates (sugars) for energy. Steps 1 and 2: Energy (calories) must be used to break down a complex carbohydrate (sugars linked together in a chain), and—see Step 3—make it available to the body as simple carbohydrates (simple sugars).

Some foods with a greater number of calories might not be nearly as likely to turn into fat as others that actually have fewer calories.

The body can only use simple sugars; this means complex sugars must be broken down into a usable form (see Figure 1.1). This process requires more energy than is required when digesting a simple sugar. The energy needed to digest complex sugars is supplied by the calories consumed. Any process that requires using energy (burning calories) will help you achieve your weight loss goal. Thus, it's easy to see how eating complex carbohydrates can lead to less fat accumulation, even though they have the same number of calories as comparable quantities of simple sugars.

The starch found in potatoes is a good example of a complex sugar. If you eat the same amount of calories in the form of a potato as you would in a glass of fruit juice, your body won't get as many usable calories because energy is needed to break down the starch. The carbohydrates in a sweet potato are even more complex, and will yield even fewer usable calories than a plain potato.

The energy needed to digest complex sugars is supplied by the calories consumed.

Simply put, *to the body*, the 200 calories in simple sugars *are not the same as* the 200 calories in complex sugars. This occurs because calories must be burned to break down complex carbohydrates into simple sugars, leading to a net caloric gain of slightly less than 200 calories for the sweet potato. Figure 1.1 illustrates the concept of using energy (calories) to break a carbohydrate chain into simple sugars that can be easily used by the body.

Some complex carbohydrates are so fibrous that they can't be assimilated by the body. Instead, they pass through the digestive tract without adding anything to the body—including calories. Celery is an excellent example of a food that contains abundant fiber that can't be adequately assimilated. As a result, you can eat celery in quantity without gaining any weight. In fact, celery requires so many calories to break down that it leads to a *net loss* of calories. Many non-root stalk vegetables have similar properties, although usually to a lesser extent than celery.

Carbohydrates are not the only food source our bodies use for energy. Other sources include fat, protein, and alcohol. A key to weight control is to understand that each of these food sources provides *different* amounts of energy when eaten in equivalent gram weights. For example, a gram of protein contains far less energy than a gram of fat.

A second important concept is that one source of food with the same number of calories as another doesn't necessarily provide the same amount of *usable* energy. For example, even though a gram of simple sugar and a gram of protein contain the same number of calories, protein requires more energy to be broken down into a useable energy form, making the actual number of useable calories from the protein less than the number of available calories from the same amount of simple sugar.

As shown in Table 1.2, 1 gram of carbohydrate or protein contains 4 calories of energy; 1 gram of alcohol provides 7 calories; and 1 gram of fat provides 9 calories. You might assume that 10 ounces of simple sugar (simple carbohydrate) will give you the same amount of energy as 10 ounces of protein. *This is not true.* Ten ounces of sugar are far more likely to end up stored as fat, because the body burns more calories when digesting protein, compared to the calories needed to digest simple sugars. *This principle is one of the keys to losing weight and avoiding an increase in fat accumulation in the body.*

TABLE 1.2 CALORIC CONTENT OF FOOD SOURCES

Energy Source	Calories per gram
Protein	4
Carbohydrate	4
Alcohol	7
Fat	9

In contrast to simple carbohydrates, a great deal of energy in the form of calories is needed to break down protein and convert it into usable energy for the body. Basically, this means that eating more protein results in less weight gain. Also, the amino acids that make up proteins are the building blocks that our bodies use to develop muscle. With this in mind, 10 ounces of protein become far more desirable than 10 ounces of simple sugars if you want to lose weight or increase muscle strength.

Eating more protein results in less weight gain.

This means that 10 ounces of sugar have more *effective* calories than 10 ounces of protein. The term "effective calories" takes into account the energy needed to convert the food into a form the body can easily use or store. Foods with more effective calories per ounce are more easily incorporated into the body and provide a greater net gain in accessible energy. For many of us, this can mean a greater accumulation of fat.

People living in developed countries often eat far too much sugar, and many older adults do not eat adequate amounts of protein. As Table 1.2 shows, fats have the most energy per gram. Ounce per ounce, fat provides much more energy than protein. Fat also contains far more energy than an equivalent amount of carbohydrate. However, more energy is needed to break down fats than simple sugars. A diet that is *low* in simple sugars is associated with burning more calories at rest— also known as an increased *basal metabolic rate*—when compared to a low-fat diet. Thus, given the same amount of calories from fats compared to simple sugars, the number of easily absorbed and accumulated calories from fats is less than with simple sugars. Additionally, a diet that is high in fat is accompanied by greater calorie expenditure when at rest. Thus, a diet of equivalent amounts of simple sugars, compared to fats, can lead to greater weight gain.

A successful weight loss program requires that we eat minimal amounts of fats and simple carbohydrates.

Overall, a successful weight loss program requires that we eat minimal amounts of fats and simple carbohydrates, and, as we get older, we should modify our diet to include more protein.

TIPS FOR REACHING YOUR IDEAL BODY WEIGHT

Here are two simple hints that will help you to achieve your fitness goals. First, *include sufficient vitamins and minerals in your diet and stay adequately hydrated.* Vitamins, minerals, and water are needed to help break down fat. If you are trying to lose weight, drinking a full glass of water before each meal will:

If you are trying to lose weight, drinking a full glass of water before each meal will have multiple benefits.

► Relieve the feeling of being hungry, because sometimes the mind doesn't make a clear distinction between thirst and hunger

► Provide a structural expansion of the stomach that also helps reduce the feeling of hunger

An adequate intake of vitamins and minerals increases the breakdown of fat and aids in the formation of muscle. Table 1.3 lists some nutrients that are often deficient in the diets of older people. Making sure your diet contains adequate amounts of these nutrients can lead to improved endurance and increased muscle mass. This is equivalent to increasing your *exercise capacity,* which can lead to improvements in overall function and even survival.

Our second hint for improved fitness is to *get sufficient sleep.* Getting adequate sleep alters the biochemicals in the body that are associated with hunger and the accumulation of fat. For example, a naturally occurring chemical in the body called *leptin* reduces hunger and decreases fat cell formation. Getting adequate sleep

Getting adequate sleep alters the biochemicals in the body that are associated with hunger and the accumulation of fat.

TABLE 1.3 NUTRIENTS LACKING IN THE DIETS OF MORE THAN ONE-THIRD OF PEOPLE OVER 65*

Folate and vitamin B complex (thiamine, riboflavin, niacin, and vitamins B_6 and B_{12})

Zinc

Magnesium

Vitamin D

Calcium

Protein

Iron

*Based on the Recommended Dietary Allowance (RDA) with 3-day food records of community-based seniors.

increases the concentration of leptins, and, ultimately, this makes it easier to lose weight.

SUMMARY

The combined forces of age and evolution have created a natural tendency for the human body to store fat. For many people, getting older is accompanied by a desire to lose the excess weight that has been gained over the years, and to improve muscle mass and strength. You can adjust your eating patterns and achieve these goals relatively rapidly. The emphasis of this book is not so much on decreasing the amount of food you eat, but rather on selecting foods that enhance fat loss and increase muscle mass. The next chapter considers practical principles based on each individual's personal goals, circumstances, and activity interests.

The emphasis of this book is not so much on decreasing the amount of food you eat, but rather on selecting foods that enhance fat loss and increase muscle mass.

Before turning to the next chapter, take a close look at Chef Speckamp's recipe on the next page. This delicious soup is loaded with protein, and it's also great for staying hydrated. Crabmeat is an excellent source of protein with very few effective calories. Maryland Blue Crabs from the Chesapeake Bay are my favorite, and they can even be purchased canned. One serving of this soup contains about 80 calories and 40 grams of protein.

Chilled Tomato Soup with Basil and Crabmeat*

Yield: 1 ½ quarts

Calories per serving: 80; Protein per 1 cup serving: 7 g

2 lbs ripe tomatoes, cored and cut into wedges

¼ cup champagne vinegar or other mild white wine vinegar

2 cups chicken stock, more as needed

½ cup coarsely chopped fresh basil

Salt and freshly ground black pepper

2 Tbsp coarsely chopped fresh mint

1 tsp Tabasco sauce, or to taste

2 garlic cloves

½ lb crabmeat (preferably jumbo lump), any shell or cartilage removed;
   canned crab can be used if fresh is not available.

1 Tbsp tomato paste

Combine the tomatoes, half the basil, mint, garlic, tomato paste, stock, and vinegar in the bowl of a food processor. Process until pureed, about 3 minutes. Refrigerate the soup and remaining basil if preparing the soup for the next day.

When ready to serve, adjust seasoning with salt, pepper, and Tabasco and process for 1 minute more. If the soup seems too thick, add a bit more stock and vinegar, if necessary.

Pour the soup into chilled bowls. Garnish with the crabmeat and remaining basil and serve.

* This soup is best in the summer when tomatoes are fresh and ripe. Don't replace fresh herbs with dry.

2

Eat and Exercise More Wisely

THE ABILITY TO ADAPT
IS A SIGN OF INTELLIGENCE

This chapter deals with general concepts about diet and exercise. Some apply to people of any age, but many are more useful and appropriate for those of us who are 50 or older. Although some of you might not be able to take advantage of them all because of a medical condition, a diet with reduced calories accompanied by increased exercise is likely to be beneficial to people with conditions such as hypertension and diabetes.

Before making any changes in your diet or exercise program, consult your physician or other healthcare professional. Talking with a physician about weight loss has been shown to increase the likelihood of success. Additionally, certain medical conditions can affect a person's ability to lose weight and might affect the foods and types of exercise they choose. Later chapters contain specific recommendations for people with a variety of medical conditions.

The principles in this book are based on recognizing the changes in your body that occur as you grow older and using that information to guide behavioral changes that will optimize your

Before making any changes in your diet or exercise program, consult your physician or other healthcare professional.

health and appearance in the short term, as well as for the remainder of your life. Following them will go a long way in helping you look better and *feel* better (and younger).

Adding Life to Our Years

As we get older, we tend to lose muscle mass, strength, and bone mass. Fortunately, we can do some things to change this. It is certainly true that a younger person who exercises the same amount as an older one is likely to develop greater muscle strength. However, we can compensate for this by exercising more, and we can certainly be in better shape than a younger person who has not exercised as much. Proper exercise is a key to improving your well-being and even to living longer. Chapter 5 is devoted to how and when to exercise for the best results.

There are many reasons to begin an exercise program. Improvements in cognition (memory), physical function, and longevity have all been linked to proper diet and exercise. Unintentional weight loss late in life can be a sign of poor health and impending illness, but *intentional* weight loss is associated with improved health and longevity. Overweight and obese women who have a sedentary lifestyle are more likely to have poor health at a younger age.

> *Proper exercise is a key to improving your well-being and even to living longer.*

To optimize the potential benefits, you'll need to combine smart exercise with smart food choices. In addition to understanding what types of food you should eat and the most advantageous times of day to eat your meals, you also need to consider how exercise affects your metabolism. Exercise continues to affect how your body burns calories long after you've done your last repetition, step, or curl.

It is also important to understand that exercise can only improve muscle strength and bone formation if your diet provides adequate amounts of protein and calcium, which are the building blocks of muscle and bone. They act in the same way as mortar does in holding the bricks of a building together.

Certain foods should be eaten soon after you exercise, in order to help your body form new muscle. Specifically, you should eat a substantial amount of protein—often 10–20 grams—within 30 minutes of completing a rigorous exercise session ("rigorous" is any exercise session that gets you breathing heavily). Protein helps build muscle and stops existing muscle from being broken down as a source of energy, because, similar to fat, muscle can be used to generate energy in the body. Many of you will choose a protein energy bar, based on the amount of protein on the package label. If you like to sit down for breakfast after a morning workout, two of the crêpes in the recipe at the end of the chapter along with an 8 oz glass of milk (preferably skim to reduce the calorie load) will provide 14 grams of protein.

Exercise continues to affect how your body burns calories long after you've done your last repetition, step, or curl.

A post-exercise protein "load" helps improve muscle strength and energy expenditure, while preventing the formation of fat. In other words, the timing of eating protein makes it easier to have a leaner, stronger body. Specific suggestions on what and when to eat are covered in Chapter 4 and in the recipes in Chapter 11.

Eat a substantial amount of protein within 30 minutes of completing a rigorous exercise session.

REDUCING FOOD INTAKE MIGHT NOT OPTIMIZE WEIGHT LOSS

Simply reducing the *amount* of food you eat will not maximize weight loss. You need to consider three additional factors.

▶ *Water* is an important part of most metabolic processes, and it accounts for most of the weight fluctuation that occurs over the course of a day. As mentioned earlier, drinking adequate water is important if you want to increase your strength and lose fat more rapidly. Plus, the stomach expansion that water produces makes it easier to avoid overeating.

► *Getting up from the table* after you sit down to a meal is often the greatest challenge. Once you leave the table, your initial battle to avoid overeating will almost always be successful. When you clean up after a meal, try to have someone help you so your mouth will not become a receptacle for leftovers! Throwing food away is better than eating it simply to avoid spoilage. While no one wants to be wasteful, it's better to throw it away than gain unwanted pounds.

► *Make sure your diet contains adequate vitamins and minerals.* Take the Recommended Dietary Allowance (RDA) or the United States Recommended Daily Allowance (USRDA) of these nutrients to help you develop muscle and bone, while increasing fat breakdown. With the exception of vitamin D, which can be given *in limited amounts* in 50,000 I.U. capsules, *avoid megadose vitamin supplementation.* Most water-soluble vitamins are excreted in the urine when excessive amounts are consumed, and high levels of some fat-soluble vitamins, such as A, D, E, and K, can be toxic or interfere with other vitamins. For example, excessive amounts of vitamin A can interfere with the beneficial effects of vitamin D on bone.

A multivitamin with minerals is sufficient for most people, with some exceptions. We now know that some nutritional requirements change as adults get older. Chapter 4 goes into more detail about vitamins and supplements. Note that most people only need a few vitamins and minerals in supplement form to meet their needs. Most healthcare providers recommend additional supplementation with calcium, to make sure that you get over 1 gram per day in divided doses. *At least* 800 I.U. of vitamin D should be taken orally per day, depending on your circumstances and sunlight exposure. Vitamin D can remain in the body for long periods of time, so this vitamin can be taken in large quantities but less frequently. Taking 50,000 I.U. of vitamin D_3 monthly is roughly equivalent to taking almost 1,700 I.U. per day (50,000 I.U./30 days). Taking a vitamin B complex supplement that includes folic acid is also important, because these nutrients are often inadequate in the diet of older individuals.

HOW MANY MEALS SHOULD I EAT, AND WHAT ABOUT SNACKING?

There is a lot of debate about whether we should eat six or more small meals throughout the day; three square meals a day (why the term "square" is used is beyond me...the plates almost always seem to be round and the food groups comprise a pyramid); or one large meal each day. One thing that seems clear is that we don't have enough information to make a confident recommendation. However, we can make some suggestions based on the available information and the principles of evolution.

As noted earlier, an exercise session should be followed by adequate protein intake. A protein supplement can be convenient and easy, such as whey protein powders that are added to a beverage, or protein bars that are low in fats and carbohydrates. Protein bars are portable and often provide about 20 grams of protein. You should have one substantial meal during the day, preferably in the late afternoon rather than in the evening. Try to avoid eating after 8 P.M., because energy levels are lower at night and eating late in the evening usually translates into fat. Of course, if you simply eat a small meal later in the evening, and your total food intake leads to a net loss in calories, you will still lose weight.

Try to avoid eating after 8 P.M., because energy levels are lower at night and eating late in the evening usually translates into fat.

MIND OVER MEALS

Knowing when and how to eat still isn't enough. You will have ample temptation to deviate from your planned eating patterns and exercise routines. Keeping busy—with both physical and mental activities—will reduce feeling hungry. It is important to respond to feelings of hunger, which generally mean that your body needs energy. Since this energy will often come from fat, if you have not taken in enough calories to satisfy hunger, it can be considered a message that you are losing fat. Still, you need to satisfy urges to eat and drink with *something*. Many snacks can satisfy hunger without providing a lot of calories. The snacks listed in Table 2.1 are relatively high in fiber (complex carbohydrates that require more energy to digest), proteins, other nutrients, and taste, but relatively low in fat-producing calories. The list is by no means exhaustive, and you will discover many other options as you incorporate the basic principles of this book into your diet strategy.

Relatively low-calorie foods are preferable, but high-calorie foods might be acceptable if these calories come from foods high in protein and fiber, or complex carbohydrates (a baked sweet potato would fit the bill as a source of protein, fiber, and starch). Unlike some diet books, *Fit At Fifty and Beyond* does not entirely exclude any foods, and no specific foods have to be included in your diet. Specific recommendations and recipes are made in later chapters, but to whet the palate, a versatile, low-calorie recipe that ranks particularly high on the taste index is given at the end of each chapter. Table 2.1 lists some foods that can help curb cravings without resulting in a dietary disaster.

As with many things in life, the toughest part is reaching your initial goal. Once you have achieved your desired weight or fitness level, maintenance requires considerably less effort.

Sustaining your new lower weight can be accomplished with a higher caloric intake than what is needed to lose weight in the first place, because your basal metabolic rate will be higher when the percentage of muscle in your body has increased. As you use this book to

TABLE 2.1 FOODS AND FLAVOR ENHANCERS THAT WILL CURB YOUR APPETITE WITHOUT ADDING TO YOUR WAISTLINE*

Mushrooms marinated in water and spices (Berkley and Jenkins), 10 calories/oz

Any vegetable marinated in vinegar or water (*not* oil) with other spices, <40 calories/cup

Raw or steamed vegetables, <50 calories/cup

Egg Beaters® with peppers, onions, etc., 30 calories/quarter cup

Salsa, 20 calories/2 tablespoons

Skim milk with Sorbet® Strawberry or Chocolate Syrup, 75 calories/cup

Special K® Cereal, 150 calories/cup with half cup of skim milk

Better'n Peanut Butter® peanut spread, 100 calories/2 tablespoons

Fat-free half & half, 20 calories/2 tablespoons

Fat-free Parkay Spray®, negligible calories per spray

Sugar-free hot chocolate, 50–70 calories/cup

Rice cakes, 50 calories each

Frozen watermelon, <50 calories per cup (despite containing simple sugars)

Frozen blueberries, about 40 calories per half cup

Sugar-free flavored gelatin, less than 10 calories/3 ounces (almost 90 g)

Lite or Fat-free Cool Whip®, 15 calories/2 Tbsp

Steamed shrimp or crabmeat, <50 calories/third of a cup

Lean meat such as chicken breast, 250 calories/cup

Two chocolate graham square with 2 Tbsp of fat-free Cool Whip® (placed in freezer), 100 calories

*See later chapters for a more comprehensive list of recommended foods, and foods to be avoided, and always remember to drink 1–2 full glasses of water as an appetite suppressant.

Once you have achieved your desired weight or fitness level, maintenance requires considerably less effort. develop a body with less fat and more muscle, you will be able to expand the amount and type of food you eat without expanding your waistline. Chapter 6 explains how you can occasionally splurge without any ill effects and—just as importantly—without any guilt!

Planning a Successful Exercise Program

We can't overemphasize how important it is to supplement your diet with exercise. If you haven't exercised in the past, you'll want to develop a routine that fits your lifestyle. Later chapters emphasize the merit of exercising in the morning. If you're not a morning person, this doesn't mean that exercise won't work for you. It only means that exercise later in the day might not optimize the effects of your workout, but it will still be very beneficial.

An exercise partner can help you stay motivated, even if your partner can't make it to every session. Having someone join you for a walk every Monday, Wednesday, and Friday means that you will be more likely to stick to your routine on those days, because now two people are counting on you—you *and* your partner. It also becomes a social experience, which often helps the time pass more quickly.

You should try to exercise at least 3 days per week. With this as the goal, many people plan to exercise 5 days a week, knowing that one or two sessions might be missed. If you make all five sessions, you will feel particularly rewarded and reduce the time needed to reach your target weight and fitness level. Detailed exercise routines are discussed in Chapters 3 and 5.

If you need additional guidance in making changes in your lifestyle, *Living SMART: Five Essential Skills to Change Your Health Habits Forever* can guide you to strategies that can help you optimize your fitness goals (see Resources).

Summary

The most successful changes in lifestyle are those that fit your own personality. Optimizing the types of food you eat and the time of day you eat will give you the best weight loss results. Exercise also should become part of your overall routine. When you need additional motivation, an exercise partner can often be mutually beneficial. Success in changing your behavior involves both mental and physical effort. The nice thing about changing your lifestyle late in life is that you will already have a good idea about what works for you and what doesn't. Now for that recipe I mentioned earlier.

By now you've probably noticed that the recipes only give total calories and the amount of protein. This is because too many people spend inordinate amounts of time computing the amount of different fats, carbohydrates, etc. in everything they eat. When you focus on maximizing strength and weight loss, you mainly need to have a general idea of how many calories you consume, stay away from simple sugars, and eat sufficient amounts of protein. Our recipes are relatively low in simple sugars, and for that reason you don't need to count carbohydrate calories. Don't get hung up on measuring amounts of fats (the *type* of fat is more important, as discussed in Chapter 4, and these recipes avoid the bad types of fat). Both fat and carbohydrate quantities have been left out of these recipes to help you avoid the temptation to focus on them.

When reviewing other recipes, shopping, or even looking at a restaurant menu, you'll want to know about the amount of simple sugars (so you can limit them), protein (knowing that you want to get your daily allotment), and calories overall (even effective calories need to be taken in moderation). In the following recipe, you have a versatile food with minimal calories, few simple sugars, some protein, and great taste. The calories are so low that you could even drizzle on a little honey without feeling guilty!

Dr. Gloth's Low-Calorie/High-Taste Crêpes

Yield: 15–20 crêpes (serves 5–10 people)

Calories per crepe: 55; Protein per serving: 3 g

2 eggs

1 cup egg substitute (e.g., Egg Beaters®)

1 Tbsp Splenda® Granular (for cooking and baking with equal measures to sugar)

1 tsp salt

1 cup fat-free half & half

1 cup skim milk

1,5 c flour

Mix ingredients.

Coat pan with low-calorie butter-flavored cooking spray

Pour just enough batter to thinly coat the bottom of pan (tilt pan back and forth until bottom is almost completely covered). Flip crepe once bubbles become visible. Cook for only another 15 seconds and serve. Makes 15–20 crêpes at about 55 calories each.

For breakfast and dessert crêpes, drizzle with honey and/or fresh fruit. Other fillings can be used for other meals. A lump crab filling is a favorite in Maryland and is very low in calories.

3

Getting Started

EAT TODAY FOR TOMORROW WE DIET— *NOT A GOOD IDEA!*

Starting a program of better nutrition and exercise is the most difficult step. The fact that you are reading this book means you recognize that you have room for improvement! However, this is only the first in a series of hurdles between the person you are now and the better, healthier, and happier person you want and need to become. If, like many of us, your initial challenge of attaining fitness through diet and exercise can be achieved simply by deciding on a program and actually starting it, you'll be pleased to know you can take many approaches to help you reach your goals.

People often embark on a major splurge in food the day or even the week before beginning a new journey down the road to dieting. This concept is steeped in tradition. Mardi Gras is a week of partying, eating, and drinking prior to the 40 days of Lent. Shrove Tuesday, the day before the beginning of Lent, is built around lots of eating before this period of relative fasting. You might have done the same thing in preparation for reading this book. For others, a splurge is simply part of the psychological preparation for making a major change in their eating habits. While understandable,

Starting a program of better nutrition and exercise is the most difficult step.

splurges usually translate into additional pounds. A brief binge might result in your needing an additional week or even month to achieve your desired weight and level of fitness. Remember, you are making a *lifestyle* change; the sooner you start, the sooner you will see results—and the easier it will be. The beginning is also an excellent time to acknowledge the many temptations and excuses that lie ahead. Make a conscious decision at the outset to find the psychological strategy to overcome them or, better still, to avoid them completely.

FROM MIND TO BODY

It is important that you see results *early* in your new program, and you need to prepare mentally for change—even a healthy one. While you can certainly achieve better fitness without it, your scale can be helpful if you use it correctly. By "correctly" we mean that it is a useful measure of *change*, not simply an instrument to measure an endpoint. In other words, don't get caught up in trying to achieve a number on a scale. You are trying to achieve a shift from fat to muscle, which can give you a much better and healthier appearance with only minimal, if any, absolute weight loss. Anyone can lose 5 pounds overnight, but most of the weight lost will be water. Such a loss might be associated with dehydration accompanied by fatigue and a less healthy appearance—especially for older adults.

> Don't get caught up in trying to achieve a number on a scale.

> With the proper mindset, your scale will help reduce temptation and be an instrument of support.

Staying focused on your fitness goal with reasonable patience will lead to lasting, healthy results. With this in mind, use your scale as a monitor of progress only when weight loss is desirable and advisable. It should be used to provide a baseline weight as well as encouragement and positive reinforcement. With the proper mindset, your scale will help reduce temptation and be an instrument of support.

Day One—The First 24 Hours

The first day of your journey to fitness starts with an evening departure. After the last meal of the day, get on the scale and record your weight. This begins the diet portion of the fitness program. From this day forward, *do not eat after 8 P.M.* except as discussed in Chapter 6 on deviations ("Falling off the Wagon…"). Go to bed early, because you'll need to wake up early for your morning workout.

Exercising in the morning is important for several reasons. First, there is little in your stomach or bloodstream in the way of energy resources, so your early morning workout will cause your body to burn up stored fat. Additionally, physical exertion places stress on your muscles, which break down to some extent. Not to worry—this process is necessary to eventually increase muscle mass.

Weigh yourself when you first get up in the morning. The difference in weight from the night before might be surprising, but it also might be encouraging. The next step is to begin your exercise routine. If you must eat first, make it a very light meal mainly consisting of protein. Whatever your initial fitness level, the basic principles will not vary. Your workout should involve some cardiovascular activity such as walking or running. These weight-bearing aerobic exercises also offer the advantage of helping to build stronger bones. Nonetheless, if you have difficulty with weight-bearing exercises, try rowing, cycling, or swimming instead.

You might be thinking, "There's no way I'm waking up even one minute earlier, and if I did, it wouldn't be to exercise—at least not until after breakfast!" While not everyone is a "morning" person, this regimen is ideal. Nonetheless, it is better to work out later than not at all. So, if this is your preference, you do have that flexibility and should not lose heart.

An additional benefit of exercise at the start of the day is that after about 20 minutes of exercising with an increased heart rate, the heart and circulation start to respond in ways that have long-term effects on overall conditioning. These cardiovascular benefits can also produce an increase in your *resting metabolism.* This means that after you have finished exercising, you will use more energy during the rest of the day, even when you are not exercising. To accomplish this, your morning exercise routine should last for at least 30 minutes, while maintaining your heart rate at about 80 percent of maximum. You don't need to continually monitor your heart rate, but you should avoid taking prolonged rest periods. You can stretch between exercises, but periods of stretching should not last longer than a few minutes.

Your workout should include some upper-body and mid-body exercises such as weight-lifting—perhaps military presses, standard curls, or some combinations of similar exercises. Specific recommendations regarding types of exercise, frequency, and duration are provided in Chapter 5. As a general rule, lift only the maximum weight that will allow you to do at least twenty repetitions without losing form. Weightlifting has been shown to be useful even in 90-year-olds, and it improves strength and reduces bone loss. Both men and women can lift weights, and it is particularly advisable for women, who might be more susceptible to developing osteoporosis as the result of bone loss. Combining weight-bearing cardiovascular exercise, such as walking, with *light* weights can help improve strength, stamina, and bone health, by helping to prevent or even reverse osteoporosis when combined with proper medical oversight and, in some cases, medication.

Weightlifting has been shown to be useful even in 90-year-olds, and it improves strength and reduces bone loss.

THE RIGHT FORM

Bureaucrats aren't the only ones who insist on using the right form! Good form is also required when exercising. The risk of injury increases with age, especially if you have gotten out of shape, which is more technically referred to as being *deconditioned.* Deconditioning can predispose you to illness and injury, so getting *back* in shape has many health benefits, including making it easier to stay in shape.

If an injury does occur, healing is slower in older adults. When you are exercising—especially as you enter your sixth decade and beyond—it is extremely important that you always pay attention in order to minimize your risk for injury.

Before running, always warm up by walking and gently stretching. Lifting should be done with the legs, while keeping your back upright and straight. *Exercise with a smooth, slow effort.* Avoid jerky motions when lifting, stretching, or doing other types of exercise, because they increase your chance of injury. Remember, it is not the *quantity*, but the quality of your effort that is important. Specific stretching, warm-up, cool-down, and other exercises are covered in Chapter 5.

> *Getting back in shape has many health benefits, including making it easier to stay in shape.*

YOUR POST-WORKOUT ROUTINE

As noted earlier, you should eat food that is low in fat and simple sugars after completing your exercise regimen. This should include complex carbohydrates and about 20 grams of protein, a little less for lighter routines and a little more for longer, more vigorous routines. Don't worry about the exact amount. The important thing is to eat some protein after exercise in order to build muscle strength. Most prepared foods have the protein content listed on the package nutrition label. On days when you exercise, your protein intake should exceed 50 grams—unless otherwise indicated by your physician or other healthcare professional. Depending on your exercise and energy expenditure, you might need to increase your daily protein intake to 60–100 grams. Exercise is usually associated with fluid loss, so drink water liberally before, during, and/or after exercise.

Visit the scale again after you complete your morning exercise. Do this daily after your morning workout. Weighing yourself at other times of the day is optional, based on whether it encourages or assists you in resisting the urge to overeat. It is generally unrealistic to expect to lose more than half of a pound in a day on average. A good goal is about 2 pounds per week.

EATING FREQUENCY

No rule states that everyone must eat three meals each day. It is also helpful to recognize that we often eat far more than our bodies need. Not every meal should be a large one. Ideally, it would probably be best to eat dinner between 4 and 5 P.M., if it is going to be your largest meal of the day. If you can't eat this early because of work, other scheduling conflicts, or choice, try to eat as soon as possible after 5 P.M., and most definitely avoid eating after 8 P.M. Dinner is a social event for many people. If you are careful about what you eat at dinner, you will probably be able to control your weight far more easily. You may have low-calorie drinks up until bedtime. Warm skim milk has a scientific basis for inducing sleep, or you might prefer rice or soy milk.

DAY TWO—ALTERNATING EXERCISE REGIMENS

As we get older, it takes longer for our muscles to recover after exercise. For this reason, you should alter your exercise regimen from day to day. On day 2, your exercise regimen should focus on different muscle groups than those you emphasized on the first day. The cardiovascular part of your workout could involve rowing, biking (including stationary), swimming, or some other kind of repetitious exercise that increases heart rate. Then, do some abdominal exercise, followed by upper body exercises different from those you did the first day; for example, switch from curls to reverse curls, or switch from an upper body to a lower body workout. Try not to focus on the same muscle

groups 2 days in a row. Even slight alterations in *Try not to focus on*
exercises are acceptable, such as shifting from *the same muscle*
regular push-ups to inclined push-ups. *groups 2 days in a*
row.

Fortunately, there are an odd number of
days in a week, which allows you 1 day off the
alternating routine. This can be either a weekday or during the week-
end. You might find that planning to exercise 7 days each week will
assure you of getting at least six workouts during the week. Barring illness or substantial injury, nothing less than 3 days a week is ever acceptable. Even on the seventh day, you might find that some physical,
recreational activity is relaxing.

Exercise raises the level of chemicals such as endorphins in the
body, which helps improve mood throughout the day. Eventually, missing the daily boost that your workout gives you will leave you feeling
"off," and your next day's workout will be even more satisfying.

Continuing Your Routine

You should continue your alternating-day routine, increasing the level
at which you exercise as your general fitness improves. You will sometimes need to make adjustments. For example, you might need to modify your routine when you are traveling (see Chapter 7). Holidays and
other alterations in your daily routine will provide minor challenges,
which you can easily overcome with intelligent preparation and some
willpower. Theoretically, increasing the amount you exercise without
changing your food intake should result in weight loss. To accelerate
reaching your fitness goals, you should simply reduce your effective
calorie intake in addition to becoming more active.

Finally, the Internet provides new ways to help you plan your exercise routines and optimize your eating patterns to help you lose weight.
One useful site is: www.lightenupamerica.org, which provides information about healthy eating and physical activities, as well as opportuni-

To accelerate reaching your fitness goals, you should simply reduce your effective calorie intake in addition to becoming more active.

ties to get involved in friendly team competition for the amount of weight lost or the amount of activity over various periods of time. Many people find that the feedback and additional motivation is helpful in reaching their weight and fitness goals.

SUMMARY

Weight reduction and improvement in fitness should involve lifestyle modification. The sooner you exchange bad habits for good ones, the easier and more quickly you will see improvement in your body and energy level. Taking the first step in any journey should be preceded by some planning, which can make the trip easier. For many people, the first step of an adventure is the most important, so start off in the right direction and know where to get the necessary supplies along the way. The remainder of this book will help you embark on your journey, with clear guideposts about the types of foods that are helpful, foods to avoid, and exercises that will optimize function and improve your overall well-being. As your fitness level improves, your overall health will also improve.

The following chapters can help make the path easier, lighten the load—both literally and figuratively—and increase the likelihood that you'll arrive at a satisfactory destination that you can enjoy for a lifetime. Your trip will likely mean getting out of the house, and simply being outside lends itself to fun exercise and fun dining.

When the weather's right, exercising outdoors seems to make workouts go faster, and they are often more enjoyable. Some of my most enjoyable cooking takes place outdoors as well. Here's a great recipe for outdoor grilling enthusiasts. Not only is this one full of taste, but it's especially good for a post work-out meal, because it is high in protein and low in calories—and even lower in effective calories.

Spicy Grilled Shrimp

Yield: 6–8 servings

Calories per serving: 93; Protein per serving: 22 g

You can make this recipe easily if you have access to Asian ingredients.

2 lbs peeled, butterflied shrimp

1½ tsp minced fresh ginger

3 garlic cloves, minced

1 tsp Tabasco sauce

1½ Tbsp rice wine vinegar

1 tsp fish sauce

1½ tsp Chinese five-spice powder

1 tsp sesame oil

Butterfly the shrimp by cutting the back lengthwise about two-thirds through, then open.

Combine the shrimp with the remaining ingredients and marinate under refrigeration for at least 1 hour.

Shake the excess marinade from the shrimp and grill until thoroughly cooked, about 2 minutes on each side.

4

Lead Us Not Into Temptation

YOUR DIET IS WHAT YOU EAT, NOT THE ABSENCE OF FOOD

The two principles involved in achieving a successful diet are to eat better food and avoid overeating. Eating less will be important for most readers, but many people lose weight just by changing *what* they eat. We often eat simply to pass the time, rather than to provide the nourishment we need. It is always more difficult to cut back when food is all around us, especially when we are not full. The challenge is to avoid temptation, so it makes sense to participate in activities that distract you from thinking about food. These activities can be physical, such as exercise, or more cerebral or spiritual, such as reading or meditating.

> *The two principles in achieving a successful diet are to eat better food and avoid overeating.*

Exercising when you are trying to lose weight is a great distraction, because it improves conditioning by burning calories, and because it does not involve eating!

Altering the quality as well as the quantity of food that you eat is important when you are trying to lose weight. Additionally, remember that you are eating to live, and not vice versa. Eat only when you are really hungry, and stop eating once your hunger is appeased—*not* after you are completely stuffed and incapable of fitting one more morsel into a belly that is ready to burst! Although this seems intuitive, it is far more challenging than it sounds, because our brains are programmed to have us store as much food as possible when it is available. You will need to adjust psychologically, which often means mentally preparing yourself to take smaller portions and limit seconds.

Rather than saying that you should not eat certain foods, focus on eating foods that are lower in effective calories and require more energy to digest, which means eating less fat and simple sugars. We emphasize this important theme throughout this book, but it doesn't mean that you can't occasionally have these foods. When you have a real craving for something that should generally be avoided, indulge, but do so sparingly.

EAT TO LIVE, BUT ENJOY WHAT YOU EAT

Eating impulsively is the downfall of many dieters. While the Biblical advice to avoid temptation in the first place might be the best advice of all, in reality it helps to have some additional strategies as a backup! The next time that temptation arises consider this: Pause and recall the last time you ate the same dish or treat, and consciously *reflect on its taste* while you re-evaluate whether it is really worth the experience, given the cost in calories. This will often help you to avoid actually eating the initially tempting treat. "Reflecting on the taste" means to mentally re-create the image of putting the food into your mouth, its texture in your mouth, and the actual taste. It also includes remembering the sensation you experienced after swallowing it.

Treats that were initially tempting probably won't seem so worthwhile after this mental exercise, and you will have avoided a costly expenditure of calories! If you decide to satisfy your desire by tasting the tempting morsel, eat only a *morsel*. Savor it and then step away. On reflection, you'll either be content with the experience, or you'll decide it wasn't worth the calories. Either way, you'll have satisfied your curiosity without doing any real caloric damage!

Plan Ahead

Eating spontaneously can easily lead to disaster. When you are very hungry, even eating at a scheduled time can lead to overeating if you aren't paying attention. Most hunger pangs stop after you eat even a small amount, and well before you feel full. By putting down your fork or spoon between bites—especially when you've come to the table famished—you'll give yourself an opportunity to actually enjoy your food as well as recognize that you aren't hungry any longer but are eating for pleasure or out of habit. By slowing down in this manner, you are more likely to stop before overeating and to stay within your caloric limits.

There are many reasons for eating. Some are *physiologic* and are needed to sustain life and maintain normal body functions; others are *psychosocial* and involve celebration, tradition, camaraderie, or even emotion.

One response to the sensation of hunger can be to eat, which is fine at the right time and in the right amount. However, if your goal is to lose weight, hunger is a beacon of success. Keep in mind that hunger reflects your body saying "I'm losing weight!" and it is a welcome sign of ongoing success. This is not to say that you should be uncomfortable throughout the process. If we advocated suffering as the way to lose weight, not many of you would continue reading! There are many ways to curb hunger pangs. For example:

When you are very hungry, even eating at a scheduled time can lead to overeating if you aren't paying attention.

▶ Hunger and thirst often overlap, so you can sometimes suppress hunger by drinking a low-calorie beverage.

▶ Another option is to exercise, because strenuous activity almost always takes away the feeling of hunger. Even if you are still hungry afterward, the impact of eating will be less after exercise.

▶ If you successfully avoid eating, exercise can be followed by a brief nap. Sleep alone often will improve energy and reduce hunger, because it helps to curb appetite and fat stores by producing beneficial changes in some chemicals in the body, such as the leptins, as mentioned earlier.

▶ Another option is to eat foods that have limited amounts of effective calories, eating only the amount needed to suppress your hunger.

▶ Sometimes trying a small taste of a tempting food item will be sufficient to stop a craving, but you must do this consciously and stop after a very small portion.

One great way to control weight is to make a conscious effort to have smaller portions and limit eating seconds. As simple as this seems, it can make a huge difference in total calories and, ultimately, in successful weight reduction. Again, the extra effort to *think* about reducing your total intake before going into the dining room or kitchen makes it far more likely that you'll be able to control your food intake. Planning in advance of a tempting situation and setting clear parameters for yourself makes it more likely you will be able to maintain your level of control.

Some restaurants now offer smaller portions of at least some entrées, including an increasing number of fine restaurants, which is very useful for those of us who would like to try some dishes without completely blowing our dietary regimen. The added bonus is that these smaller portions are usually less expensive as well! Even relatively big eaters have been pleasantly surprised to find that they are satisfied and don't need to consume as much food to feel that way.

Eating often serves a psychosocial function as much as it does a need for physical survival. Consider how eating and behavior interact. Many studies have shown that people are more likely to eat more if the meal occurs in a social setting. Certain holidays—such as Thanksgiving—are actually *linked* to eating. Some people also eat more in certain circumstances, such as being in a depressed mood. By considering the influence of different situations on eating, you can either avoid them entirely or plan in advance to cope with them. By considering those aspects of eating, and re-evaluating the link between eating and various situations and events in your life that are associated with overindulgence, you'll be far more likely to curb your eating at such times.

> *Eating often serves a psychosocial function as much as it does a need for physical survival.*

TYPES OF FOOD

As noted earlier, some foods—such as celery—can be eaten without much concern about weight gain. These foods are generally either very low in calories, or the available calories are quite complex and provide fewer effective calories, or both. Other foods that are generally so low in calories that you can eat them without concern include most stalk vegetables (broccoli, asparagus, and cauliflower), as well as other vegetables that are typically served as appetizers (peppers, carrots, cucumbers, and mushrooms). Additionally, these foods are high in the complex carbohydrates called *fiber*. High-fiber foods, including cereals (grains, etc.), have also been linked to reductions in the risk for cardiovascular disease. Most vegetables in the legume family, which includes beans and peas, contain useful amounts of protein, but some also contain more calories as vegetable fats and are not as useful for unlimited consumption.

In addition to raw or steamed vegetables that can be eaten in relatively large amounts without substantially contributing to your effective calorie count, good snacking choices include sugar-free flavored gelatins (which can be combined with fat-free whipped topping for a guilt-free snack or dessert), fat-free popcorn, and rice cakes. Tea, coffee, broths, and artificially sweetened beverages are also on the list, and sugar- and fat-free hot chocolate is a good treat for people who like chocolate.

Foods that are high in protein and low in fat and simple sugars include shrimp, crab, some fish, and lean meats (chicken, venison, ostrich, bison, certain cuts of beef, and most wild game). Although relatively high in fat content, the high proportion of protein in salmon makes it a good example of a relatively high-calorie food that is acceptable, because of the energy needed to break down the protein and beneficial fats. Some fats are essential, and deep sea fish is an excellent choice; it is also one of the few natural sources of vitamin D.

This is a good time to discuss fat intake. Not all fats are the same. There are *essential* fats, and there are fats that should be avoided. Many products are touted as "fat-free" as a means of attracting diet-conscious people who associate fat with gaining weight. This concept has more to do with marketing than science. Hopefully, by reading this book you now realize that 100 calories of fat actually provide fewer effective calories than 100 calories of simple sugars. By the end of this chapter, it should be clear that the right type of fat might also be much better for you.

Not all fats are the same.

Although people in Western cultures who consume large amounts of saturated fat have relatively high rates of heart disease, people in countries that consume relatively large proportions of monounsaturated fat (as in olive oil) and polyunsaturated fat (as in fish) tend to have a low incidence of coronary heart disease. Avoiding fat is probably related to the fact that much of the fat eaten in the United States and Canada is from red meat and is therefore saturated fat. Saturated fat has been linked to an increase in low-density lipoprotein or LDL, which has been associated with what many people call "bad cholesterol." Monounsaturated and polyunsaturated fats result in more high-density lipoprotein or HDL, which is related to what is commonly called "good cholesterol." It is the ratio of LDL to HDL that determines risk for cardiovascular disease. Low LDL and high HDL create a ratio linked to a reduction in heart disease.

A low-fat diet that reduces monounsaturated or polyunsaturated fats and increases carbohydrates results in the production of another cardiac risk substance called *triglycerides*, while also reducing HDL. This worsens the LDL-to-HDL cholesterol ratio and increases triglycerides, making the risk for heart disease even worse!

Another type of fat is *trans-unsaturated* fatty acids (trans-fats). These artificial fats are man-made by the partial hydrogenation of liquid vegetable fats (oils). This process causes the oils to solidify. The resultant trans-fats are found in margarines and many baked goods and fried foods. Trans-fats raise LDL and triglycerides at the same time they reduce HDL. Thus, they create the worst of all conditions for developing heart disease.

Foods that are high in monounsaturated and polyunsaturated fats include poultry, fish, various vegetables, and many commonly ingested nuts. Deep sea fish are particularly high in omega-3 fatty acids, which seem to be extremely beneficial in preventing heart disease. They might also be helpful for other health reasons. When you have the option of choosing foods containing these beneficial fats versus equal caloric amounts of carbohydrate-laden options, the food with the greater composition of fat would be better for your diet and overall health.

Trans-fats raise LDL and triglycerides at the same time they reduce HDL. Thus, they create the worst of all conditions for developing heart disease.

BEVERAGES

Fluids are also a source of nutrition and calories. Some beverages are particularly good choices. For example, skim milk is an excellent source of calcium and protein, and it is as good as whole milk but with far fewer calories. If you are lactose-intolerant—a very common issue in older adults—similar benefits can be obtained from drinking soy milk or skim milk containing Lactaid®, an enzyme that breaks down the sugars that produce symptoms of lactose intolerance.

People who don't like skim milk will find that this preference is simply based on experience, and it can be changed after a month or so of using it instead of whole milk. You can get the same result more slowly and perhaps more easily by switching in stages—to 2 percent, 1 percent, and then finally to fat-free milk.

Most fruit juices have no protein, are abundant in simple sugars, and

Fluids are also a source of nutrition and calories.

should be drunk only sparingly. If you drink fruit juice, it should be unsweetened and calcium-fortified. Unsweetened or artificially sweetened teas and coffees have relatively little nutritional value, but they can be enjoyed without concern about calories.

ALCOHOL

Many people enjoy beverages containing alcohol. If you consume alcohol, do it sparingly, because there are almost as many calories in an ounce of alcohol as in an ounce of fat, and these calories are more accessible to the body than calories from fat. Mixed drinks that combine alcohol with simple sugars or high-fat creams are very high in calories and should be avoided. Use substitutes for sugar and cream instead. For example, use artificially sweetened tonic water in a gin and tonic, or make an excellent Brandy Alexander with low-calorie, fat-free half & half.

Here is a recipe for eggnog that was developed by my favorite cardiologist (and brother), Dr. Sean Gloth, based on our grandfather's recipe. It offers the taste of this festive holiday family favorite, but with far fewer calories and without the artery-clogging elements of regular eggnog:

Dr. Sean Gloth's Egg Nog

10 oz fat-free half & half

2 oz brandy

2 oz rye, bourbon, or mixed blend whiskey

4 oz rum

1 cup of Splenda® Granular sweetener (for baking and cooking)

1 cup of Egg Beaters®

Mix all ingredients in a blender and serve chilled. This recipe makes 5–6 drinks with fewer than 200 calories each and with far more protein and other nutrients than most alcoholic beverages.

Lower-calorie choices are also available for beer and wine. Most light beers contain 90–100 calories per 12 oz. Michelob Ultra® is an attractive option because it is low in both carbohydrate and fat. Amstel Light® has the same number of calories with about twice the number of carbohydrates and protein as Michelob Ultra®, making the trade-off with carbohydrates and proteins a reasonable option as well. Most other light beers are similar in their effective calorie content, so taste can be the determining factor in your choice. Even with "light" beer, the effective calories mean that most people should not have more than one or two in a day.

Wines contain calories from sugars in the grapes, as well as their alcohol content. Nevertheless, wine is an important component of some meals. White wines generally contain more simple sugar than red, but you can make your choice based on taste because the difference is relatively small. Aim to have no more than one glass of wine with a meal.

The bulk of calories in most spirits come from the alcohol content when no mixers or sugars are used, or when low- or no-calorie substitutes are used. Moderate alcohol intake—up to 1.5 ounces of alcohol per day—may have some health benefits. Calories and other issues should discourage you from additional indulgence.

CHANGING NUTRITIONAL REQUIREMENTS AND SUPPLEMENTS AS YOU AGE

Dietary needs change with age, and some nutrients need to be increased. For example, the calcium requirement for men *and* women jumps from about 1,000 mg a day before 50 years of age to 1,200–1,500 mg a day at age 50 and beyond. The Required Daily Amount (RDA) of vitamin D has been increased to 600 I.U. per day for people over 70, and the National Osteoporosis Foundation has recommended an increase to 800–1,000 I.U. per day for people 50 and older (compared to the 400–800 I.U. per day recommended for younger adults). Unfortunately, at the same time as these requirements increase, most people's intake of these nutrients actually decreases.

This makes it easy to understand why many healthcare professionals recommend nutritional supplementation for seniors. While "mega-dose" vitamin and mineral supplementation can be wasteful—or worse, toxic—a standard multivitamin with minerals each day is probably reasonable for most people who might be getting insufficient amounts in their daily diet.

Dietary needs change with age, and some nutrients need to be increased.

Calcium and vitamin D intake might still be inadequate for many older people even if they take a multivitamin, because few foods contain sufficient calcium and vitamin D to satisfy dietary requirements. Although vitamin D can easily be obtained through exposure to sunlight, many of us don't get enough. Therefore, we recommend adding 500 mg of elemental calcium three times a day and at least 600 I.U. per day of vitamin D for older adults.

Even with calcium supplementation of a gram per day, people who lose weight will also lose bone if they don't incorporate some weight-bearing exercise into their regimen. This emphasizes the importance of increasing exercise when losing weight. It also makes it clear that a good diet—with or without supplements—is not adequate, by itself, to optimize fitness and health.

Many older adults require 800–2,000 I.U. of vitamin D daily to achieve adequate vitamin D status. Vitamin D is a fat-soluble vitamin that can actually be taken infrequently; for example, once monthly, as long as the dose averages to the daily 800–2,000 I.U. per day. While vitamin D status is very dependent upon age and sunlight exposure, most people do well with 100,000 I.U. of vitamin D only once monthly. This dose actually averages out to a little more than 3,000 I.U. on a daily basis.

There are two types of vitamin D—vitamin D_2 and vitamin D_3, whose technical names are *ergocalciferol* and *cholecalciferol.* Either formulation is fine, when taken on a daily basis. Taken once monthly, 50,000 I.U. capsules of vitamin D_3 might make a more prolonged contribution to vitamin D stores and consequently to health and strength, although information is limited as to how this relates to the type of vitamin D used.

Regardless of which form of vitamin D you take, it is associated with many health benefits, including reducing some forms of pain, decreasing falls and fractures, and improving strength. Most folks recognize that vitamin D helps build strong bones, but its many nonskeletal benefits might be even more important. For example, in addition to the benefits noted above, vitamin D relieves the symptoms of seasonal affective disorder (SAD), a form of depression associated with a lack of sunlight and, therefore, more prevalent in winter.

Diet As a Lifestyle Change

Don't think about changing your diet as simply restricting the food you eat, but as a change in your eating patterns and behavior that will optimize your overall health and fitness. Keep in mind that your goal is to achieve a desirable protein-to-fat ratio, and to eat only a minimum amount of simple sugars. Your overall plan should include participating in other activities, including physical activity, which will help keep your mind off of food. If you spend more time in activities that don't involve eating, you will become more productive, make a greater contribution to society, and enhance your personal growth. Later chapters

Don't think about changing your diet as simply restricting the food you eat, but as a change in your eating patterns and behavior that will optimize your overall health and fitness.

on exercise include recommendations for how and when to exercise, as well as suggestions for other activities that will enhance fitness.

SUMMARY

The primary message in this chapter is to stay in control of your eating. Slow down and savor each bite. If it helps to physically put your spoon or fork down between bites, then do so. Before indulging in something that tempts you to deviate from your healthy eating plan, create what might be called a "pre-eating" experience, which means visualizing the food in your mind *before* actually eating it. Imagine taking it into your mouth; imagine its texture and taste; and even imagine swallowing it. Then, if you still feel it is worth the calories, have a small taste but limit the portion. Smaller portions are a good idea, in general, and will have a measurable impact on weight loss over time. Some key guidelines include:

▶ Complex carbohydrates are preferable, especially those high in fiber content.
▶ Stick with monounsaturated and polyunsaturated fats, especially omega-3 fats.
▶ Drink more water.
▶ Incorporate more activities into your schedule, including regular exercise.
▶ When you drink alcoholic beverages, minimize the high caloric impact by avoiding the high-calorie mixers or simple sugars that are added to many mixed drinks.
▶ Vitamin supplements in the form of a daily multivitamin might be useful, but additional calcium and vitamin D supplements are warranted as we get older.

The recipe that follows is also a great one for the grill, and it takes advantage of some of these key guidelines. It combines complex carbohydrates with rich omega-3 fatty acids in a meal that is low in effective calories and high on the delectability scale! Add a nice chilled glass of pinot grigio (115 calories for a 5.1 fl oz glass), and you can settle in for an evening of contentment.

Grilled Bass with Fennel, Balsamic Vinegar, and Basil Oil

Yield: 4 servings

Calories per serving: 280; Protein per serving: 50 g

4 small fennel bulbs, tough outer layers and feathery leaves removed

6 Tbsp balsamic vinegar

1 tsp olive oil

2 Tbsp basil oil or olive oil

Salt and freshly ground black pepper

4 sea bass or striped bass fillets (about 7 oz each), preferably from the whole
   fish; any white fish may be used if bass is not available

Prepare an outdoor grill or preheat a grill pan over high heat until very hot, about 3 minutes.

Split the fennel bulbs in half lengthwise and brush with the basil oil or olive oil.

Place the fennel on the grill about 9 inches from the heat source and cook until just soft, turning several times, about 10 minutes; or add to the grill pan and cook over high heat until soft, about 10 minutes. (If the fennel seems to be charring too quickly, reduce the heat to medium.)

Five minutes before the fennel is done, place the fillets on the grill, skin side down, or remove the fennel from the grill pan when done and add the fillets. Cook the fillets for 3 minutes and rotate them about 45° to create an attractive crosshatch pattern. Cook 2 minutes longer; turn, and cook 2 minutes more on the second side.

Remove the fennel and fillets to plates. Sprinkle with the balsamic vinegar and olive oil. Season with salt and pepper and serve.

5

How and When to Exercise: Exercises for Older Adults

SMART EXERCISE FOR OLDER ADULTS

Along with smart eating should come smart exercising. "Smart" exercising means doing the type of exercises that maximize outcome while minimizing the risk for injury. The type of exercise you do can affect many areas of your body, contributing to far more than just increases in mass and strength in the muscle groups that you use during exercise. The right types of exercise can improve your overall cardiovascular health and even increase the amount of bone deposited in your skeletal system, thus lessening the risk of osteoporosis. Resistance exercises—exercises using weights—will improve the strength, mass, and quality of your muscle tissue.

The aging process is associated with a decrease in bone and muscle mass of about 1 percent per year, and a decrease in conditioning or *functional reserve*. However, exercise can be considered almost a "miracle" intervention that can minimize much of this effect. Depending on the intensity of training, the absolute difference can be as much as one-third. Studies in 90-year-olds have shown that improvements in

> *"Smart" exercising means doing the types of exercise that minimize risk for injury and maximize outcome.*

strength and muscle mass are possible even quite late in life. Exercise also has a positive effect on longevity, cognition, mood, and balance— which is especially important in reducing the risk of falls.

Repetition—the number of times or "reps" that you do a specific exercise—is important if you want to improve your cardiovascular health. Weight-bearing exercise is the key to reducing bone loss and improving muscle mass, and your exercise routine should include exercises with heavier weights. "Heavier" is, of course, relative. Your choice of weights will vary greatly depending on your age, sex, and general health.

Before beginning any exercise program, it is important to be sure you have no medical problems that might make some types of exercise risky. Have a brief discussion with your doctor, nurse practitioner, or other healthcare practitioner before undertaking any new exercise regimen, especially a strenuous one.

FINDING TIME TO EXERCISE

Some people think they don't have time for exercise. This is simply not a good excuse. When you're exercising, you're not spending time eating, and a little less eating would be a good thing for most of us. More importantly, it is a matter of priority and time management. Ask yourself how important health and fitness is to you. If it is not important, you will be far less likely to succeed in making the necessary lifestyle changes. If you *do* want to be healthier and maintain your optimal weight—and presumably that's why you are reading this book—then you'll make the effort. The time commitment doesn't have to be excessive, and the extra time you spend will be more than worthwhile. Ideally, you need to create a daily schedule that includes about an hour of exercise.

There are many ways to exercise that will fit nicely into your daily schedule, even before you decide to carve out time specifically for a formal exercise routine. Here are some things you can do that will contribute to your fitness and—in some cases—actually save you time:

▶ Stop waiting for elevators and start using the stairs. You'll get to your destination sooner, and you'll have burned some extra calories as well.

▶ Avoid double parking or parking in an illegal spot just to be closer, even if you're only going to be somewhere for a minute. By making the effort to park in a legitimate parking space, you'll not only avoid inconveniencing someone else, you'll benefit from the extra steps—calorically speaking! Better still, park in a space farther away, where there are few other cars. If you pick a space in a lighted area where there will be no cars next to yours, you will get extra exercise, and you'll also avoid having someone opening their door into your car. That will keep your car looking better and even help its resale value.

▶ Walk to locations that don't absolutely require driving. Many places a half mile or even a mile away take less than 15 minutes to reach on foot. Walking will likely take no more time than driving, and it might actually save time while providing great exercise.

▶ When walking from your car to your office or other building, take the scenic route, especially if there is an option among multiple entrances.

▶ Do your own lawn chores and housework, and if you can, shovel your own walkway/driveway after it snows.

▶ Walk your shopping cart to the cart corral or back to the store.

▶ Take trash to the curb, and always walk to a trash receptacle with your garbage rather than leaving it in a more convenient place.

▶ Wash and wax your own car.

By being actively courteous, you're not only making the world more pleasant for others, you're burning calories as well! So leave the single parking space in the front row for someone else. Save electricity and take the stairs. All the while, your good conservation of resources will result in a better looking and better feeling you!

MAKE YOUR EXERCISE ROUTINE
FIT YOUR PERSONALITY

Many of us find that exercising is easier in a group setting. If this describes you, the camaraderie, socialization, and mutual motivation of group exercise classes will help stimulate you to participate. There are many ways to do group exercise. You can join a gym or fitness center, where such classes are usually led by a fitness instructor. Your local "Y" or senior center might offer classes, sometimes at no or minimal charge. If you're a good organizer, you might set up a small group that meets regularly in members' homes or at a local community or church hall. One of the advantages of exercising in a group situation with an instructor is that you can try a variety of classes to see which ones you like, and vary them to achieve optimal fitness. For example, you may find that yoga, tai chi, Pilates, or other types of exercise make a nice balance to those emphasizing aerobics and workouts with weights.

Some people prefer to exercise alone. If this is true for you, having exercise equipment at home will be helpful. You'll need to get into a routine of exercising at the same times during the week. This approach requires a bit more personal motivation, but it has the luxury of accommodating your schedule and saving travel time.

Many people prefer to work out with others some of the time and alone at other times. This might mean that there are certain days/times when you join a partner or group, but you work out alone on the other days/times. Alternatively, you might choose to join someone for part of your routine, but go solo for the remainder. This can provide motivation, camaraderie, and socialization, while at the same time accommodating a desire for solitude during part of your exercise routine. For example, you might start by walking or running with a partner or group, and then return home for the remainder of your exercise program. This type of arrangement can motivate you to get started—which is usually the most difficult part of exercising—and it might be a bit safer as well. It also allows you to have a partner who is at a different level of conditioning and for each of you to work on the type of exercises you prefer for as long as you'd like.

In addition to the exercise program that we provide in this chapter, many exercise tapes are available that can help you achieve optimal fitness. Some of the best ones are listed in the Resource section.

CARDIOVASCULAR EXERCISE

Depending on your current exercise capacity, you can choose from a variety of exercises that promote cardiovascular health. Walking is a good way to start if you are just beginning an exercise program or are starting again after a long period of not exercising. You can gradually increase both the distance you walk and the pace. Walking also is a good weight-bearing exercise that will help improve bone health as well as reducing overall body fat. Other cardiovascular exercises include swimming, rowing, cycling, and running. These exercises can quickly get you breathing faster and increase your heart rate. As a rule, you need to keep your heart rate up for at least 20 minutes to have a significant effect.

Exercises that improve *cardiovascular* health involve many repetitions with either no weights or lighter weights. If you use weights, select ones that allow you to do a minimum of 20 repetitions comfortably; optimally, you should do 50 more for a cardiovascular effect. As with all exercises, good form is more important than how much weight you lift or how many repetitions you do.

MUSCLE MASS

Improving muscle mass and working on body definition and tone usually involves some resistance or lifting heavier weights. Although some people use weights they can lift a maximum of 10 times, older adults should use a weight that can be lifted 10–20 times, with caution again about maintaining form and avoiding strain that can lead to imbalance or instability. You will get far better results by maintaining good posture and overall form than if you use a particular amount of weight or number of repetitions as a target. Good posture refers to keeping your back straight and shoulders back. Focus on the targeted muscle groups. If your back starts to get out of alignment, or you start to sway or jerk to move the weight, then you've reached your maximum and you should end that set. Not only will your strength and muscle mass improve more rapidly by maintaining good form and posture, but you will minimize your risk of injury as well.

You will get far better results by maintaining good posture and overall form than if you use a particular amount of weight or number of repetitions as a target.

These types of exercises usually involve free weights or exercise equipment for resistance training. The specific exercises you select will depend on the area(s) you most want to emphasize. For example, if your goal is better shoulder definition, you might focus on military presses, bench presses, or calisthenics such as push-ups.

BONE HEALTH

Weight-bearing exercises improve bone health by reducing the bone loss that typically occurs with aging. Resistance training also benefits bone health, whether done on machines or with free weights. Walking is also helpful, because of the weight shifting that occurs with each step you take. Exercises such as swimming or cycling, which do not involve any or much weight-bearing, have much less effect on bone density.

As discussed earlier, you need to provide nutritional support for your body when you exercise, especially by eating sufficient protein to improve muscle mass. For most people, this means at least 55 grams of protein each day, some of which should be eaten within half an hour of a good workout. Calcium intake is also important because it enhances bone formation and health. Older adults need more than 1,200 mg of calcium in divided doses—no more than 500 mg at a time for optimal absorption.

The *shifting* of weight seems to be almost as important as the *amount* of weight you lift. Subtle vibration (even 10 minutes a day on a low-magnitude vibration plate) is associated with improvements in bone mass, which should lead to greater resistance to fracture.

Mixing Repetitions

By increasing and decreasing weight through each cycle, mixing repetitions might help you get more general benefit from your exercise. One option is to do a cycle of increasing and then reducing weights. With this technique, you first use a moderate weight, then a heavier one with fewer repetitions, then a lower weight, and finally a very low weight. This can be an intense workout, but it often leads to more generalized improvements in a relatively short time.

Specific Exercises for Specific Areas

Upper Body

A variety of exercises can be used to improve shoulder strength and definition. If no weights are available, you can do standard push-ups or half push-ups, as shown later in this chapter, depending on your ability.

Pull-ups and chin-ups can also be very effective for the upper arms and back. Many people can't do these exercises, but machines that assist with them can help you get to the point where you can do them independently.

Lower Body

Simple walking is an excellent exercise for your legs. Other worthwhile exercises include stair climbing, running, walking in a pool, and simply sitting in a chair and straightening the legs individually and alternately. Additional workouts can include using weights, either free weights or one of the many varieties of resistance exercise equipment available. Partial squats, as shown later in this chapter, are also useful. Full squats (when your thighs actually touch your calves) can be particularly hard on the knees, and they are not recommended. Squatting no further than 90 degrees should be more than adequate for building up your leg muscles and improving balance. Back leg kicks, also shown later in this chapter, can also be helpful, particularly for toning up the buttocks muscles.

WHEN TO EXERCISE

Ideally, as discussed earlier, you should exercise in the early morning if at all possible, but exercise can be done any time. It's preferable to exercise before a meal, because eating something that is predominantly protein within the first half hour after exercising is the most helpful in reducing the loss of muscle protein and providing the protein needed to build muscle, tone the body, and burn stored fat. You need to maintain adequate hydration when you exercise, and it's particularly helpful to keep a bottle of water with you throughout your exercise regimen.

Give exercise a high priority in your life. Although some specific times might be more desirable than others, in the grand scheme it is simply important to exercise while you are losing weight. As we get older, the frequency of exercise does not need to be as intense. Exercise involves the breakdown and repair of muscle fibers, which can take longer in older adults. As a result, missing one day of exercise is quite okay. On the other hand, prolonged periods of inactivity are much more devastating in terms of loss of strength for older adults. An 85-

year-old person who is bed-bound for a week will need more than a month to recover the losses in strength and function that result from the period of inactivity. Because of this, you need to do *some* kind of exercise even when recovering from a minor illness.

You might occasionally find yourself unable to do some exercises because of injury, inflammation of an arthritic joint, or some other condition. However, exercise has been shown to reduce pain in almost every study ever done, so you need to take advantage of this benefit. Although pain can sometimes prevent you from doing certain exercises, there might be others that won't cause pain. Doing these exercises might even help reduce pain, and they will help you maintain your overall strength and function.

FORM FIRST

When exercising, always remember that attention to form is one of the most important factors in the success of your exercise program. Good form includes good posture, balance, and rhythm. Jerking motions, imbalance, erratic movements, and excessive weight or strain can make you injury-prone. An injury can be devastating—and it is also a quick way to derail a successful diet and exercise program.

Never lift with your back—and don't bend over with your spine curved when lifting anything. Always lift up using your leg and abdominal muscles, while maintaining your balance and erect posture.

Always remember that attention to form is one of the most important factors in the success of your exercise program.

The saying, "No pain no gain," is counterproductive as we get older. We might also say, "New pain, no gain," referring to the loss in function that occurs when you have a painful injury. Rather, focus on patience, doing a good routine while paying attention to form, and gradually increasing the number of repetitions and the amount of weight you lift. The exercises described here are recommended for all ages, but they are particularly useful for people who are 50 and older. The suggested variations are based on individual levels of conditioning and ability.

EXERCISING AWAY FROM HOME

You'll need to think about exercises that can be done when you don't have your own exercise equipment or environment, because there will be times when travel interferes with your regular exercise routine. This topic is covered in more depth in Chapter 7, but it's worth mentioning a few points here.

Many hotels have excellent fitness facilities. You might even be able to have a more intense workout than normal if you try some equipment that you don't normally use. If an exercise facility isn't available—or you're not comfortable using what is available—take heart. You can accomplish a lot without ever leaving your room. You can easily do sit-ups, push-ups, Pilates, and other calisthenics in your room. You can also use various items found in most hotel rooms as weights, and there are other creative ways to work in some basic exercise while you travel, as discussed in Chapter 7.

SPECIFIC EXERCISES

These exercises provide a comprehensive stretching and weight-bearing program. *You should consult with a physician or other health care professional before starting this or any other program so that you can modify exercises as needed.* We have called attention to exercises that are not recommended if you have osteoporosis of the spine or other medical conditions.

> We have called attention to the more difficult exercises. Do *not* attempt these unless or until you are at a fitness level where they can be done safely.

Warm-up and Cool-down Exercises

The first part of your routine should involve an easy, fluid set of warm-up exercises to allow your muscles to acclimate to the more rigorous part of the routine. This process will probably help reduce injury as well. Warm-up and cool-down exercises usually don't use weights, but rely more on light calisthenics. Walking at a slow pace with longer strides is always good as either part of the warm-up or cool-down routine. The first exercises described below can serve as a good warm-up. Some of the stretching exercises might be useful as part of a warm-up set or to cool down at the completion of your exercise routine.

Step Calves Workout

Stand on a step with your weight on the balls of your feet. Extend up as high as you can then slowly let down as low as you can while maintaining balance. If balance is an issue, we recommend using a step with handrails. Repeat for 10–20 repetitions.

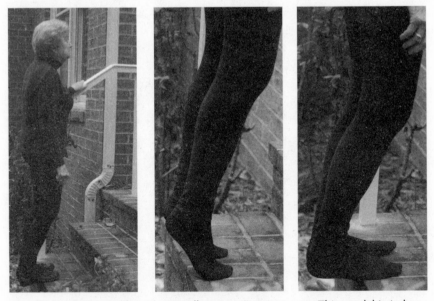

STEP CALVES WORKOUT. This is an excellent exercise at any age. This model is in her 80s. Note the handrail for stability.

Stretching

Many people believe stretching is an important component of an exercise routine. The argument is compelling for improved flexibility and contribution to injury reduction with the use of smooth and gradual stretching exercises. The key in stretching is to move slowly without undue strain or any type of jerking that might cause an injury. Stretching is used both as part of the warm-up process as well as the cool-down routine. Some preferred stretches are illustrated below.

Side Knee to Head

While lying on your back, bring your straightened leg up to as close to 90 degrees as you can. Then, turn to the side opposite the raised leg and continue to bring that leg as close to your head as you comfortably can. This is often a preferred exercise for cooling down rather than as a warm-up.

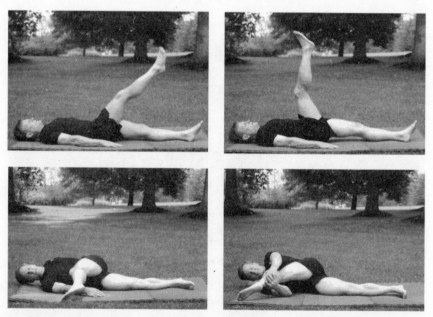

SIDE KNEE-TO-HEAD STRETCH. Various flexibility levels will allow greater or lesser stretch. A smooth continuous motion is the key here, as demonstrated by the author, who is in his 50s.

Seated Single Leg Head to Knee (Advanced)

This stretch is for those of you who are in moderate to advanced condition. Sit on the ground with both legs straight out. Then bend one knee so that your heel is next to your buttocks. From this position, bring your head as close to the other knee (with the leg still extended) as is comfortable. Count 20 seconds and switch to the other side.

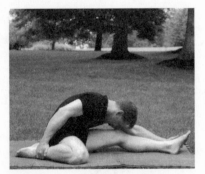

SEATED SINGLE LEG HEAD-TO-KNEE STRETCH. A smooth continuous motion applies to this stretch as well.

Legs over Head (Advanced)

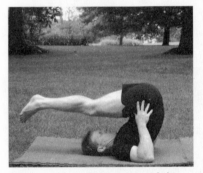

LEG-OVER-HEAD STRETCH. *Avoid this exercise if you have osteoporosis of the spine, as it increases pressure on this area.*

This is another stretching exercise for people in moderate to advanced conditioning, who do not have osteoporosis or other reasons to avoid such exercises. Lie flat in the supine position and raise both legs together and as far over your head as is comfortable. Hold for 20 seconds and repeat. If you're less comfortable with this exercise, try the head-to-knee stretch that follows.

Head to Knees

Simply sit on the ground with both legs extended in front of you and slowly bend your head toward your knees. Again, only stretch to a point that is comfortable. If you can't touch your toes, grab behind your thighs, knees, or calves (with time, you should see improvement). Hold this for 20 seconds, then relax and repeat.

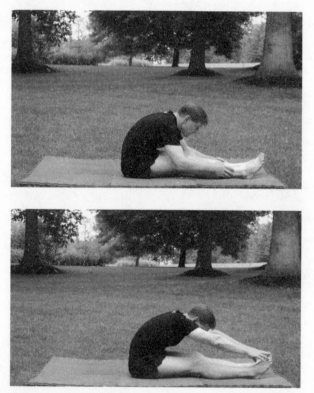

HEAD-TO-KNEES STRETCH. *Avoid this if you have osteoporosis in the spine.* Gently stretch to the point closest to knees and hold for a 20-count while pulling toward knees with hands clasped around ankles, calves, knees, or thighs, whichever is most comfortable.

Groin Extension

Sit on the ground with your legs as far apart as you can comfortably get them. Slowly bend your head toward your left knee and hold for 20 seconds, and then do the same with your right knee, while keeping both knees on the ground. Finally, bend your head toward the ground in the middle for another 20 seconds.

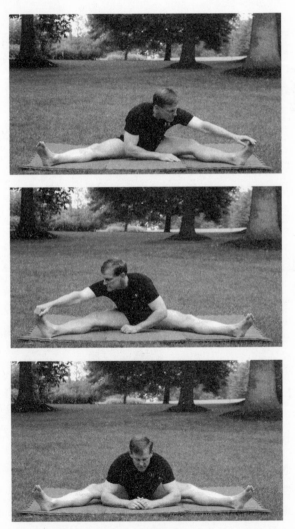

GROIN EXTENSION STRETCH. *Avoid this if you have spinal osteoporosis.* This stretching exercise is done with legs as far apart as possible.

Overhead Arm Stretch

Extend both arms as high over your head as you can. While reaching your arms up, bring your hands as close together as possible. If you can, touch and interlock your fingers while straightening at the elbows. Hold for 10 seconds.

Upper Arm Extension/Flexion

This simply uses a fixed structure to help provide resistance while you stretch your upper arms as illustrated. This allows the pectoralis muscles in your chest to stretch as well.

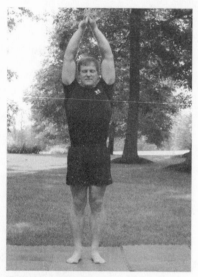

OVERHEAD ARM STRETCH. The stretch comes from extending the arms with the fingers interlocked overhead.

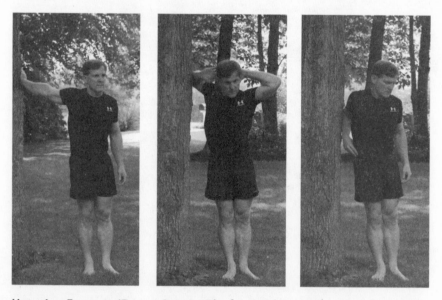

UPPER ARM EXTENSION/FLEXION STRETCH. The force in this exercise comes from leaning into an immovable object, like the tree in this photo.

Lower Extremity Extensions

These are two different stretch exercises. Figures A and B are done with the back heel remaining fixed to the ground while you stretch your calf. Figures C and D release the heel and provide more stretch for the upper leg muscles. Figures C and D require caution, with more strength required the lower you go. Again, only go to a level that is comfortable for you, and be careful not to strain or overstress your knee.

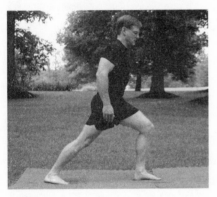

FIGURE A

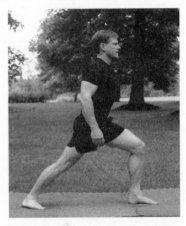

FIGURE B

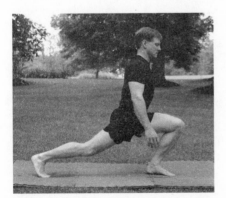

FIGURE C

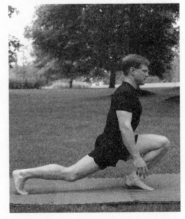

FIGURE D

LOWER EXTREMITY EXTENSION STRETCH. This stretch can be done with support of a rail if your legs are not particularly strong or if balance is an issue.

Toe Touches (As Close to Toes As You Can Go)

This stretch also needs to be geared to individual ability. It is not necessary to actually touch your toes—just lean forward in the direction of your toes while maintaining your balance. The movement needs to be smooth; hold the lowest position for a few seconds before slowly straightening up. This stretch is usually best done as a cool-down exercise.

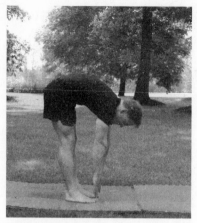

TOE TOUCHES STRETCH. Avoid this exercise if you have osteoporosis of the spine. Gently reach for the toes, but don't go beyond a comfortable distance. Hold at farthest reach for a 20-count.

Split (Very Advanced)

Many people cannot safely get to the point where their hands can reach the ground in this stretch. *Unless you have some support from a rail or other sturdy fixture, you might want to skip this stretch until your flexibility allows you to do it easily and safely.* This is generally an exercise for cooling down rather than one done at the beginning of your exercise routine.

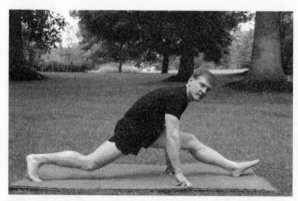

SPLIT STRETCH (ADVANCED). Consider doing this next to a fixed bar or other support to reduce risk of injury.

Partial Squats

Stand with your feet shoulder-width apart, and then flex your knees and extend your arms straight out in front of your body. Keeping your heels on the ground, try to squat down while maintaining balance, but go no further than the level at which your upper legs are parallel to the ground. As noted earlier in this chapter, going beyond this point is too hard on the knees.

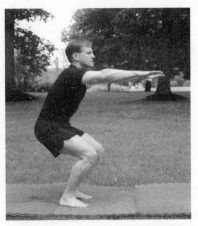

PARTIAL SQUAT FOR STRETCH, WARM-UP, OR COOL-DOWN. From a standing position with feet shoulder-width apart, squat down until thighs are about parallel to the ground.

Back Leg Kicks

Put your hands and knees on the ground as illustrated in Figure A. Then kick one leg back and extend it as far as possible while extending the

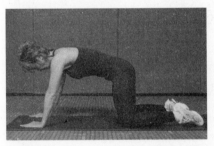

FIGURE A

opposite arm forward as shown in Figure B. Note that your back should remain straight throughout this exercise. Continue alternating between left and right for 20 repetitions.

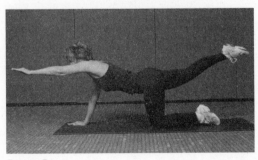

FIGURE B

BACK LEG KICKS STRETCH, WARM-UP, OR COOL-DOWN. Note that the model (Olivia Haley, Ms. Senior America 2008) gets good extension raising her leg back and up as far as possible.

Walking Arm Flexion/Extensions

This is a good warm-up exercise that you can do while walking. Start with both arms straight out in front of you with your fingers extended, and then bring your hands to your chest while making a fist. Next, extend your arms to each side while extending your fingers again. Bring your arms back to your chest while making a fist again, and then return to the original position with your arms and fingers extended in front of you. Do 50 repetitions.

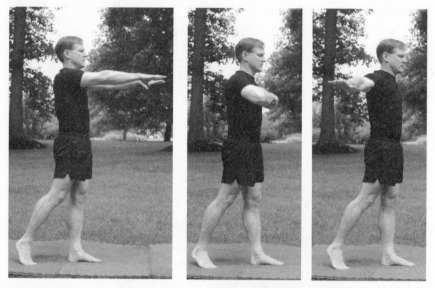

WALKING ARM FLEXION/EXTENSION STRETCH, WARM-UP, OR COOL-DOWN.

Balance exercises using Tai Chi and similar programs are also very helpful as an alternate-day workout or as a warm-up. Good instructional videos are available on Tai Chi online at http://www.taichiforseniorsvideo.com/. Two very good DVDs for beginners are *Tai Chi for Older Adults* by Paul Lam and *Tai Chi Exercises for Seniors* by Bob Klein.

EXERCISES FOR STRENGTHENING

Push-ups

If you haven't exercised for a while, you might want to start by doing half push-ups (also called "knee push-ups") as shown in Figures 5.15a and b. Allow your knees to rest on the floor, and then push up as with a regular push-up.

Push-ups can be done in multiple sets, maximizing the number that you can do, or as a single set. These are excellent exercises that work the deltoids and triceps in your upper arms, as well as the muscles of your back, neck, and abdomen.

Knee Push-ups

This exercise is good for beginners or people who are unable to do regular push-ups for any reason. If you have a shoulder problem, or other

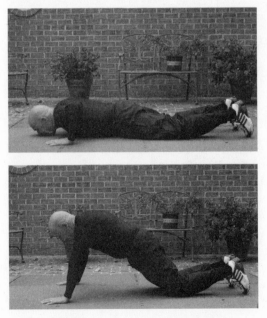

issues that make regular or knee push-ups difficult, do standing wall push-ups (similar to regular push-ups, but done against a wall instead of on the floor).

KNEE PUSHUPS. These are easier than standard pushups, but still good for arms, back, and chest.

Standard Push-ups (Somewhat Advanced)

These push-ups are done by lying face down on the ground with your legs together, and with only the bottom of your toes touching the floor. Place both palms flat on the floor and push your hands against the floor, while pushing the rest of the body up. Keep your back straight throughout the exercise. Go up until your arms are fully extended, and then return until your chin touches the floor, while keeping the rest of your body off the surface

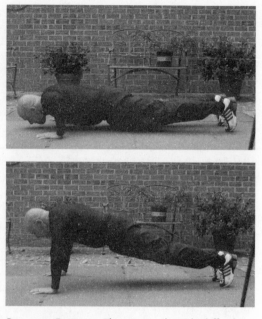

STANDARD PUSHUPS. These are relatively difficult, but are great for the chest, arms, back, abdomen, and legs. Despite being in his mid-80s, he makes this look easy!

until you are finished. Regular push-ups are for people in average to good condition.

Inclined Push-ups (Very Advanced)

These are for more advanced exercisers, and should be done keeping your back straight, either on an incline or with your feet up on a step. The higher the step the more difficult this exercise becomes.

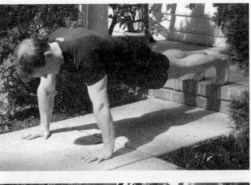

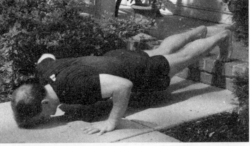

INCLINED PUSHUPS (ADVANCED). These are very difficult, but if you can handle 50 or more standard pushups, the added difficulty of inclined pushups can allow you to get a great workout with fewer repetitions.

Sit-ups

You can do a variety of sit-ups depending on your strength and flexibility. Because of the strain that can be placed on the back with other variations, the following are the only types we recommend for older individuals.

Partial Sit-ups for Beginners

Lie on the ground with your hands behind your head and your knees flexed. Push your lower spine toward the ground, but do not raise your shoulder blades off of the ground. Twenty of these should be a good initial goal.

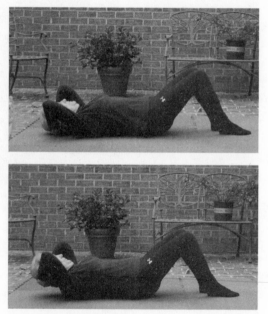

PARTIAL SIT-UPS. This is a relatively simple exercise that helps build the abdominal muscles. Note that this model in her 80s only lifts her head and starts to lift her shoulders, contracting her abdominal muscles without lifting her back off the mat.

Parallel Sit-ups (Advanced)

Start in the same position as with partial sit-ups, but instead of placing your hands behind your head, extend your arms parallel to your upper legs (knees up and feet flat on the floor). Raise your upper body, keeping your arms parallel to your upper legs until your elbows are at the height of your knees; repeat until you start to become fatigued. Twenty of these is a good initial goal.

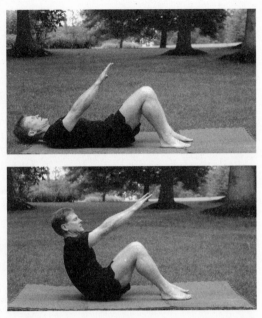

PARALLEL SIT-UPS. This exercise is so named because the arms remain out and parallel to the thighs. It is not necessary to bring the shoulders any higher than the height of your knees.

Inclined Sit-ups (Advanced)

This relatively difficult exercise is done on an incline. The key is to have your knees flexed and something (or even someone) holding your knees down. Then, while keeping your back straight, bring your chest toward your knees. Perform this exercise slowly, if possible, for a better and more difficult workout. Again, 20 is a good initial goal.

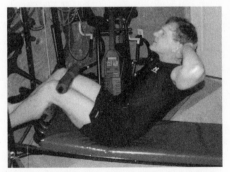

INCLINED SIT-UPS (ADVANCED). Try to keep your back straight while doing this relatively difficult exercise.

Exercises with Weights

When working with free weights, it is important to use a weight that is comfortable, regardless of what specific exercise you are doing. For some of the exercises that follow, you might be comfortable with only a bar (without any weight attached). Some people will not be able to use a standard weight bar, at least not at first. Using rods or even a 1-inch hollow pipe from the hardware store may be adequate for you, at least at first.

Military Presses

This type of exercise is commonly done by men, but many women can benefit from doing it, too, but using lighter weights or even just a bar. It can also be done with two dumbbells. However, this requires a bit more care, because lifting two weights simultaneously requires greater coordination and provides less stability.

Keep your back straight and lift with your legs—*not* your back! With your feet about shoulder-width apart, bend your knees (not from your waist) to the point at which you can reach the bar. Look straight ahead and stand up. Once you are standing erect, bring the bar up to your shoulders and then over your head. Return the bar to shoulder level and extend again over your head. Choose a weight that is comfortable for 20 repetitions and that allows you to retain good posture with fluid movement.

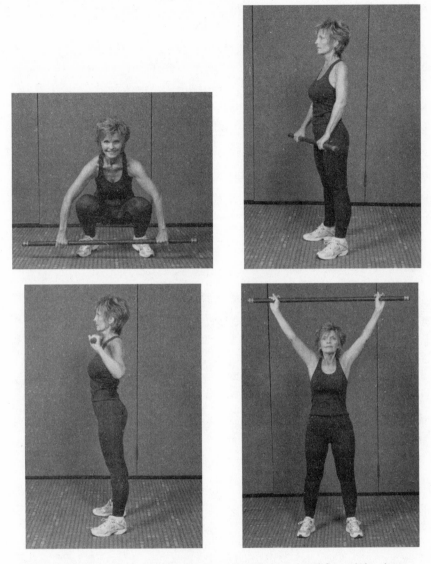

MILITARY PRESS. Note how Ms. Senior America (Olivia Haley) lifts with her legs while keeping her back straight. Use a weight that is comfortable for 20 repetitions, even if it means only using the bar.

Military Press Variation (Very Advanced)

This is done exactly like the version shown earlier, but instead of return-ing the weight to the shoulder position in front of your head, bring it down behind your head. This is more difficult and will require either fewer repetitions or less weight. Note the difference in weight compared to the prior examples for the standard military press. Working out with weights offers the advantage of appealing to every age and strength because of the ability to add or decrease the amount of weight based on comfort and ability. As one gets stronger, the number of repetitions will increase, then eventually the amount of weight can be increased to get back to 20 repetitions, and the cycle will repeat as you continue to get into better shape.

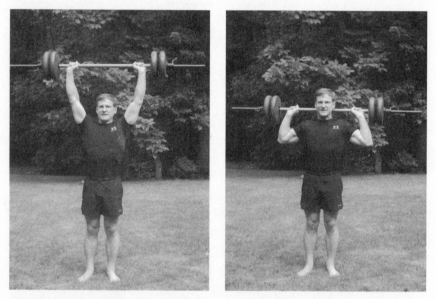

MILITARY PRESS VARIATION. This differs from the standard military press. Here the bar comes down *behind* your head.

Military Press with Dumbbells

Start with each weight on the ground, to the outside of your feet, so that you can grab them easily with your arms by your side. Again, lift with your legs and keep your back straight. Bring both weights to shoulder level simultaneously. From this position, lift both weights over your head, and then return to shoulder level and back to the overhead position repeatedly. Remember, this requires a bit more coordination and has less support than raising a single bar, so you might not be able to lift half the weight in each arm as the full amount that can be lifted in a military press using a single bar with weights.

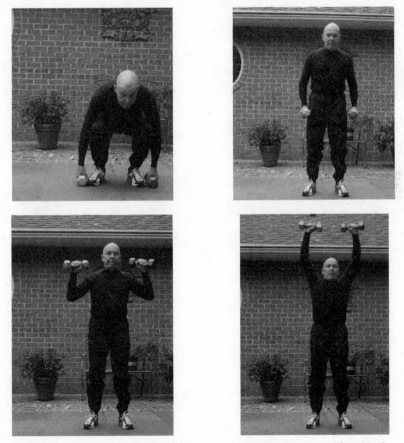

MILITARY PRESS WITH DUMBBELLS. Good form and a weight that is comfortable for you remain most important when exercising with weights.

Standard Curls with Bar (Advanced)

These exercises are great whatever your level of strength. Use a weight that is appropriate and maintain good posture. You can use a straight bar, add weights to both sides as appropriate and comfortable, or you can use a single barbell (dumbbell) type of weight and exercise one arm at a time. Either way, keep your shoulder and upper arm in position as you flex at the elbow.

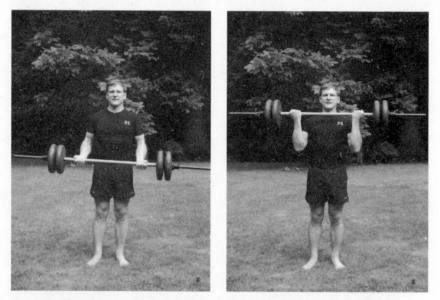

STANDARD CURLS USING A BAR. Form is far more important than the amount of weight. Use a weight that you can comfortably curl 20 times. Do *not* attempt to use the heavy weights shown here unless you are in top condition.

Dumbbell Curls

Note how the elbow stays in position and the back remains straight.

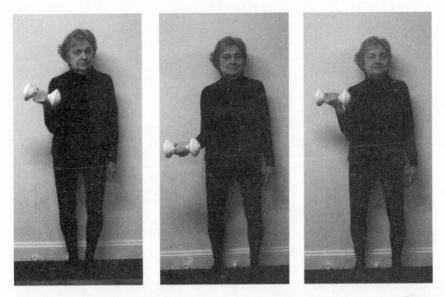

DUMBBELL CURLS WITH ONE WEIGHT. Even in your 80s, this is a good exercise. Notice how the model keeps her elbows fixed in position. This can be done with one or two weights simultaneously, as illustrated next.

Dumbbell Curls Using Two Weights Together

See Figures 5.26 a through 5.26c.

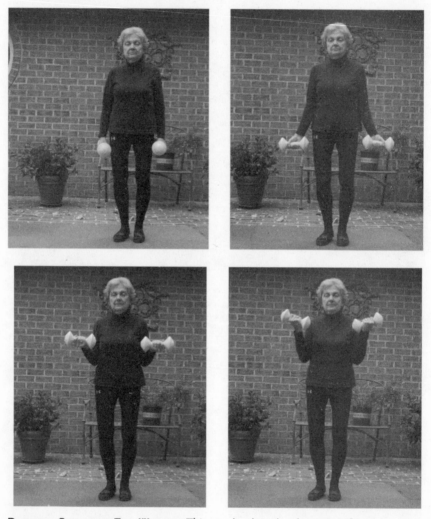

DUMBBELL CURLS WITH TWO WEIGHTS. This can be done by alternating from one arm to the other.

Reverse Curls

These are similar to standard curls, except the weight is grabbed from above the bar; again, note the erect back and fixed elbow.

Wrist Curls

These exercises use weights that are usually lighter than for regular curls. Again, use the weight that is

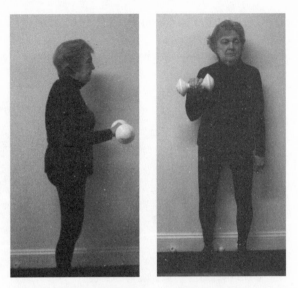

REVERSE CURLS. This is performed with the same principles as standard curls, but using a grip from above.

comfortable for 20 repetitions. Many older women will find 2–5 pounds more than adequate for this exercise, depending upon the number of repetitions.

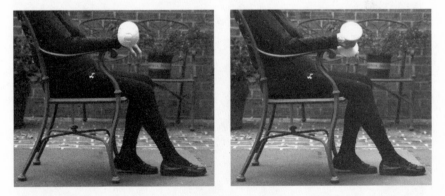

WRIST CURLS. Grab the weight from below with palm facing up. Keep your arm on the chair arm. If your chair doesn't have arms, do this exercise with your arms resting on your thigh.

Reverse Wrist Curls

The hand position here is the same as for the reverse curls exercise described earlier.

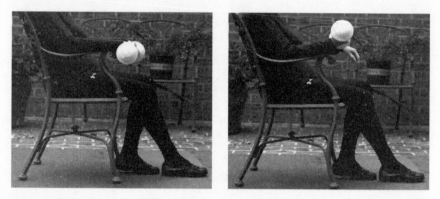

REVERSE WRIST CURLS. Just like standard wrist curls, but grab the weight from above.

Pull-ups (or Chin-ups) (Very Advanced)

Grab the overhead bar with both hands and knuckles facing out. Pull up your own weight until your chin passes the bar. This is for moderate to

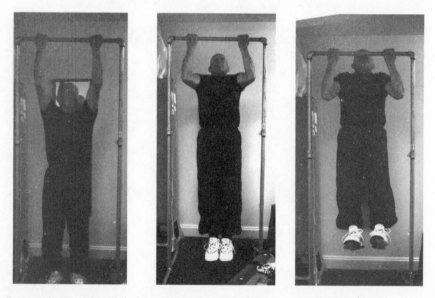

PULL-UPS OR CHIN-UPS. With this exercise, the palm of your hand is facing you.

advanced individuals, because many people cannot do this exercise without special equipment found in many gyms that allow partial weight support while doing the pull-up or chin-up.

Reverse Pull-ups (Not Illustrated)

These are similar to the pull-ups illustrated above, except that the grip is reversed. Grab the overhead bar with both hands and knuckles facing toward you. Pull up your own weight until your chin passes the bar. This is also for people with moderate to advanced levels of strength and conditioning.

Straight-Arm Pullovers

These exercises can be done by people at all levels. Even people in very good shape who are unaccustomed to these exercises will find that they can lift only light weights, or even just a bar in this exercise.

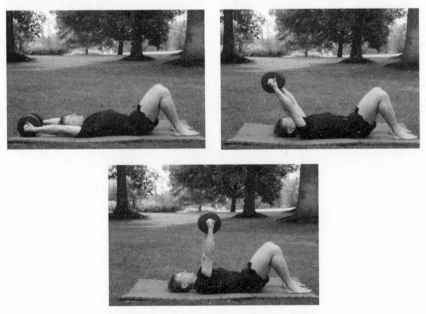

STRAIGHT-ARM PULLOVERS. This exercise is a good one for the back when using light weights.

Back Arm Extensions

Take a single weight and hold it in your hand with your arm fully extended over your head. Flex at the elbow, lowering the weight behind your head. Return the weight to the original position and then repeat until you start to become fatigued.

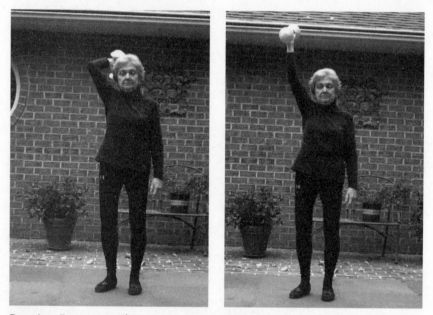

BACK ARM EXTENSIONS. This exercise is great to tone up the triceps behind the arm. Notice how the model here (in her 80s) keeps her arm and elbow stable during the exercise.

TABLE 5.1 HOW SOME OF THE EXERCISES IN THIS CHAPTER AFFECT DIFFERENT PARTS OF THE BODY

Areas Affected	Exercises
Neck	Sit-ups, Push-ups
Back, Shoulders	Military Press, Back Arm Extension, Curls, Pull-ups, Chin ups, Lateral Extension
Chest	Push-ups, Straight-Arm Pullovers
Biceps (Upper arm)	Curls
Triceps (Upper arm)	Back Arm Extensions, Push-ups
Deltoids (Upper arm)	Push-ups, Lateral Extensions
Forearms	Curls, Pull-ups/Chin-ups
Abdomen	Sit-ups
Legs	Walking, Running, Step-ups, Squats

After exercising, you body will need a meal that is high in protein, which provides the building blocks of muscle. The recipes that follow fit the bill (one for a large group dinner and one for breakfast after the morning workout).

Beef Tenderloin with Blue Cheese and Herb Crust

Yield: 10 servings

Calories per serving: 366; Protein per serving 42 g

10 5-oz portions of filet of beef

1 Tbsp parsley, chopped

1 cup white bread, crusts removed, toasted

1 Tbsp chives, chopped

½ cup blue cheese

Pinch cracked black peppercorns

Crumble all ingredients, except beef, together by hand to form coarse paste.

For each serving: Dry-sear one filet in a sauté pan. Transfer the meat to a rack in a roasting pan. Coat one side of each medallion with a portion of the crust mixture and roast in a 350°F oven until cooked to the desired doneness.

Crustless Quiche

Yield: 4 servings

Calories per serving: 160; Protein per serving: 13 g

4 slices bacon, chopped

¼ onion, chopped

1 tsp garlic, chopped

1 cup milk

1 cup Egg Beaters®

½ cup biscuit mix

½ cup cheese, Swiss (reduced fat)

1 small zucchini, shredded

1 small tomato, diced

1 tsp salt

½ tsp pepper

Preheat the oven to 375°F.

Cook bacon until crisp and all the fat has been rendered. Drain on paper towels to remove excess fat. To the bacon fat remaining in the pan, add onion and garlic, sauté until translucent. Let cool.

Mix all of the ingredients together.

Pour into a glass pie pan and bake for 25–30 minutes.

6

Falling Off the Wagon So It Doesn't Hurt

IF AT FIRST YOU DON'T SUCCEED: STRATEGIES TO PREVENT LAPSES

We all know that specific circumstances and special times of the year can tempt us back into old habits. Being mentally prepared and physically avoiding some of the worst situations can go a long way to keeping your willpower in top form so you can remain successful, fit, and feeling good about yourself.

The period between Thanksgiving and New Year's Day is notorious for disrupting an established lifestyle. Estimates vary, but commonly about 7 pounds are added to body weight during this period. Fortunately, many people successfully lose the weight they've gained once the holidays are over. This type of weight gain is usually manageable; the pounds will come off as you get back into your usual diet and exercise routine. It is helpful to understand this response to changes in diet and activity, because

Many people successfully lose the weight they've gained once the holidays are over.

it means that we can establish a new routine with minor modifications that can lead to additional positive changes in weight and strength.

Of course, it is best to avoid gaining weight in the first place, which involves establishing the right frame of mind and then using this mindset to stay on course, as we discussed in earlier chapters.

This is a good place to elaborate on the mental preparation that is needed. Most of us know our most likely downfall situations. For example, if you know that every Thanksgiving you'll be confronted by your favorite apple crumb pie (that no one in the world has ever been able to duplicate), you have two options. First, you can avoid the dessert—which is not likely to be an acceptable option. The second option is to establish a routine in your mind before you attend the party or dinner. It's the same as the golfer or field goal kicker who visualizes the shot or kick in his mind before ever stepping up to the ball. Creating a mental visualization can help you follow through with the same motion when it counts.

First, imagine being offered the eggnog, the holiday cookies, or the mashed potatoes with gravy. Establish in your mind how it will taste. Satisfy yourself that it just isn't worth the extra miles of walking or hundreds of sit-ups you would need to do in order to undo the damage done by the additional calories. Imagine avoiding these foods. Ideally, this means visualizing avoiding reaching for the dish, as well as having it offered and declining. Then imagine what you *will* consume—the lean turkey, the green beans, or the fresh cranberry sauce. This doesn't mean you can't enjoy a few splurges. Just recognize in advance what is acceptable and stick with your plan. Saving up for one splurge is actually helpful in cutting down on other distractions.

In addition to psychological preparation, physically avoiding temptation is also helpful. For example, remember that when you get up from the table after a single helping of dinner, you will experience complete satiation within minutes. This is a good physical strategy—removing temptation or removing yourself from the temptation. Remaining at the table makes temptation greater and should be avoided. Walking into another room with a cup of coffee or helping to clear the table are excellent ways to avoid overeating while still participating in the social aspects of the occasion.

When you get up from the table after a single helping of dinner, you will experience complete satiation within minutes.

If someone insists on giving you half of the remaining pie she made especially for you, take it home wrapped and put it in the freezer immediately. You can thaw it out when others are around to help eat it and dilute the caloric explosion. The advantage of using the freezer is that the pie will be out-of-sight—and out of mind. Additionally, the tempting pie will take time to thaw out before it can be eaten!

MINIMIZING DAMAGE ONCE A LAPSE OCCURS

Once you make a decision—conscious or not—to eat food that you will probably regret in the morning, you can do a few things to minimize the impact. While eating the first few bites, try to focus on the texture of the food as well as its taste. This will help to make the trip worth the destination. In other words, really enjoy it, or—perhaps—recognize that it isn't as spectacular as you had anticipated. Either way, you will genuinely appreciate the food. Additionally, it will force you to slow down and "smell the chocolate sauce," so to speak. This will prevent you from smothering yourself with chocolate kisses, and it might allow you to savor *one* without gobbling down the handful that you envisioned. Then step away from the food while enjoying the first morsel, in order to prevent yourself from eating too much of it.

In all likelihood, a one-time splurge won't cause much damage and can even be planned. You do need to make sure that your body doesn't adjust to the availability of calorie-laden foods, thus improving the efficient absorption of energy from them, which translates into additional accessible calories and fat.

DEALING WITH THE AFTERMATH OF CALORIC CATASTROPHES

The day after a major splurge, it is important to return to a focused and disciplined mindset. If you *really* overdid it, you are likely to be less hungry the following day. Listen to your body. If you aren't hungry, don't feel obliged to eat, and be sure that you consume sufficient fluids, especially water. This will help reduce hunger, increase your body's ability to burn fat stores, and help maintain your energy level, because dehydration is associated with fatigue.

It is also important to get right back into your routine. That means you need to do a good workout and be careful about what you eat. Be particularly good, rather than trying ease back into your efforts gradually. Intensely focus on this the first day after a splurge. Psychologically, you'll be tempted to be a little less stringent. The sooner that you get back into your routine, the more likely that one day of splurging will have little overall effect.

JUMPING OFF THE WAGON: PLANNED DEVIATIONS

Another approach is to pick specific days during which you are allowed to spoil yourself a little bit. It's best if you have a good workout on the days you allow yourself a planned indulgence. On those days, go for the chocolate-peanut butter ice cream or the blueberry pie. Even then, plan ahead and splurge in a controlled fashion—have a *slice*, not the whole pie! You'll often find that a smaller portion will satisfy your craving and only do half the damage.

Again, savor each morsel—really *experience* the indulgence. If it isn't as delicious as you expected, remind yourself of this the next time you're tempted. As we grow older, our tastes and desires change. You might only desire your favorite sweet from childhood because of its link to another time, but now you no longer experience the same pleasure it once gave you. This is one reason why it seems as if no one can duplicate some of the delicacies you remember from your childhood. Don't worry; there will be many other pleasant experiences to add to those distant memories!

Pick specific days during which you are allowed to spoil yourself a little bit.

The other important part of a planned occasional indulgence is that it can't come too often. More than once a week is probably too often. The other point to remember is that alcohol can lower your control. We say this only to emphasize the importance of moderation. Many liquors and wines enhance both the taste of food and the dining experience, but drinking too much at one time will quickly add calories and lower resistance. A glass of red wine offers many health benefits, but drinking half the bottle will probably negate these benefits. This can be a disaster when you are trying to maintain a healthy lifestyle.

One of the other reasons that the occasional indulgence is acceptable—and doesn't cause much of a problem for maintaining your weight—is that the absorption of any food is modified based on what you usually eat. This means that some of the foods you have avoided for a long time will not be absorbed as well as they would be if they were eaten regularly. For example, if you have not been eating much fat, and then eat a meal with a high fat content (and calories), your body will not be used to absorbing the higher amount of fat. This occurs because the cells lining your digestive tract have adapted to allow the positioning of certain molecules and receptors that absorb fat. This won't happen if you simply have an occasional meal high in fat. However, once the body adjusts to a higher fat level, it will be better prepared to absorb fat. This is also why you shouldn't repeat splurges too close together.

Planning a splurge also gives you the opportunity to do a bit extra in anticipation. This might mean exercising for a bit longer or eating a bit less. All of this will allow you to enjoy your splurge and assuage any guilt that you might otherwise experience.

Summary

Mental preparation is important, especially when going somewhere where food will be a central focus. Picture in your mind encountering and avoiding high-calorie foods. Slowly savor the foods that you eat, especially those that are loaded with calories. Remember to get back into your regular exercise and eating routine quickly after a splurge. If you are going to splurge, do it in a controlled fashion and with a good exit strategy!

The following recipe is a great way to start back on the right dietary path and has great flexibility—it's good for breakfast, lunch, or dinner. Beyond the few simple sugars in the milk, most of the calories in this dish require energy to become available to the body in a usable form. Hence, there will be slightly fewer effective calories than what is given in the "Calories per serving" count. Knowing that the effective calories here will offset some of the total calories, you'll find this dish even more enjoyable.

Spinach, Mushroom, and Goat Cheese Tart

Yield: 4 servings

Calories per serving: 245; Protein per serving: 7 g

Pie Shell

½ cup all-purpose flour

3 Tbsp unsalted butter, cold

1 Tbsp vegetable shortening, cold

1½ Tbsp ice water plus additional if necessary

Filling

1 Tbsp olive oil

½ cup white mushrooms, medium size

1 cup spinach leaves, packed fresh, trimmed, washed thoroughly

½ cup Egg Beaters®

⅓ cup whole milk

⅓ cup goat cheese, crumbled

Preheat oven to 425°F.

In a bowl, with a pastry blender, or in a small food processor, blend together the flour, butter, shortening, and a pinch of salt until the mixture resembles meal. Add water and toss until incorporated, adding additional water if necessary to form dough. Pat dough onto bottom and one half-inch up the sides of a 7½-inch tart pan and bake in the bottom third of oven until set and pale golden, about 7 minutes.

While shell is baking, in a skillet, sauté mushrooms in oil over moderately high heat, stirring 2 minutes. Add spinach and sauté, stirring, until wilted and tender, about 2 minutes. Remove skillet from heat and season spinach mixture with salt and pepper. In a small bowl, whisk together Egg Beaters® and cream.

Sprinkle goat cheese over bottom of shell and arrange spinach mixture on top. Pour cream filling mixture over spinach and bake tart on a baking sheet in the middle of the oven 15–20 minutes. Reduce the temperature to 350°F and bake until set, about 10 minutes.

7

Maintaining Your Diet and Exercise Lifestyle When You Travel

MAINTAINING NUTRITION WHILE AWAY FROM HOME

Getting the right types of food when you are eating out or traveling definitely requires some thought and planning. Fortunately, most restaurants offer light fares that are lower in calories yet nutritionally healthy. Even when you are conscientious about selecting the right foods from a menu, when you get back on your scale at home you might find that you gained weight. Take heart—most or all of the weight gain is due to the higher salt content of foods in restaurants and the fluid retention it produces. The weight will disappear without effort after a few days of your usual attention to diet and exercise. Many chefs have trouble cooking without adding salt—usually using far more than many of us use at home.

> *Most restaurants offer light fares that are lower in calories yet nutritionally healthy.*

Of course, when you travel, you might be exposed to new delicacies that you'll want to sample. As long as you're careful, you can try most new culinary experiences without doing any real damage. This means eating foods low in effective calories and—when confronted with something that doesn't meet your culinary criteria, but presents a dining experience far too tempting to turn down completely—opting for a predetermined number of bites, preferably two or less! Savor the taste and appreciate the experience, but don't get carried away. You are not required to be wasteful. Many restaurants are willing to offer sampler selections. This allows a few people to share without accruing excessive calories individually. Even if such a selection is not available, take advantage of sharing desserts anyway. Many restaurants will split a selection and serve it on separate plates. Finally, don't be afraid to request that your treat be packed to go. Depending on the durability of the selection, some treats can be savored again the next day when your calorie count totals can better afford it.

It is also helpful to keep a few protein bars handy when traveling. Since you can't always find healthy food, they will provide a great form of sustenance, and they are particularly helpful after a workout if a good protein source is not readily available within about 30 minutes. Without recommending anything specific, try to get a bar that has an acceptable taste, more than 15 grams of protein, fewer than 200 calories, and fewer than 5 grams of simple sugars.

HYDRATION

It is also a challenge to stay hydrated while traveling, especially because it is harder to carry liquids on planes these days. You can buy water after passing through security to supplement what you will be given on the plane. Having water available the morning after you get to your hotel can be a challenge. One tip is to fill your ice bucket prior to going to bed. A lot of the ice will melt overnight, and you'll have refreshing ice-cold, usually filtered water when you wake up the next morning. (A word of caution is in order. Many hotels in the United States filter the water going to the ice machine, but that is often not the case elsewhere, and ice in some less-developed countries can be a source of dangerous bacteria. It is usually easy to tell if a separate filter is used for the ice machine by looking for it hanging from the water supply line.)

It is important not to be tempted by sweetened sodas or other beverages because of their high simple sugar and effective calorie content. Although most fruit juices have greater vitamin content than standard carbonated beverages, they are generally loaded with simple sugars and should be drunk sparingly or avoided. Vegetable or tomato juice might be a more practical substitute. Water—carbonated or not—with a squeeze of lemon remains a top choice for staying hydrated while traveling. Tea and coffee might have other merits, but both have natural diuretic qualities and are not great hydrating liquids.

Skim milk has more protein and fewer effective calories than many other commonly available beverages. As discussed in previous chapters, the calcium and vitamin D that skim milk contains are also important factors to consider, because both are usually deficient in our diets as we get older.

EXERCISING WHILE AWAY FROM HOME

Many people have a great exercise routine at home, but have difficulty maintaining any semblance of a routine when traveling. Exercising while on the road is especially important, because controlling dietary intake might be more challenging. Fortunately, many hotels have fitness areas with excellent exercise equipment. However, the quality and selection of equipment varies tremendously, as does the cost of using it. Some hotels include the cost of a fitness center in the room price, while others can be quite expensive. Regardless, effective and enjoyable exercises can be done using "equipment" found in most hotel rooms. Even outside of your room you can "stair climb"—not using a machine, but actually

> *Exercising while on the road is especially important, because controlling dietary intake might be more challenging.*

climbing stairs. This is an excellent workout for your legs and cardio-vascular system, and it's free.

Some exercises, such as push-ups, partial push-ups, wall push-ups, 90-degree squats, snap-ups, parallel partial sit-ups, and stretching, can be done in your room (see Chapter 5 for illustrations). Curls and triceps exercises can be done using the (clothing) iron in your hotel room as a weight, or a chair as illustrated below. These items can be used for other exercises as well. Always inspect any in-room equipment before using it for purposes other than those for which it was designed. Using tables or chairs, for example, for support or to lift is only recommended when stability and safety can be assured. *Never risk an unnecessary injury, simply because you wanted an additional exercise opportunity.*

Chair curls are very dependent on your strength level and the type of chair in the room. Use common sense and the principle expressed earlier of not lifting anything that you can't lift comfortably with good form at least twenty times.

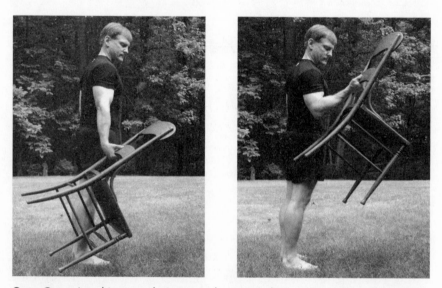

CHAIR CURLS. Iron biceps and triceps workout (not shown). Do curls as illustrated with chair above, but use a clothes iron.

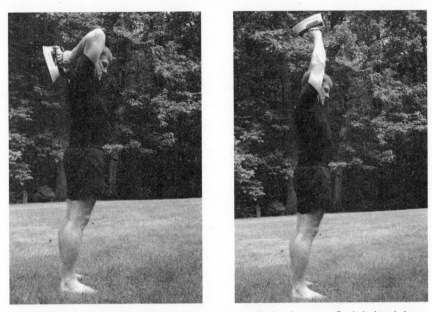

TRICEPS EXTENSION. Triceps extensions can help with that hanging flesh behind the arm. It requires good posture and can be done with one arm or two together, depending on the weight. This excellent exercise can be done with the clothes iron.

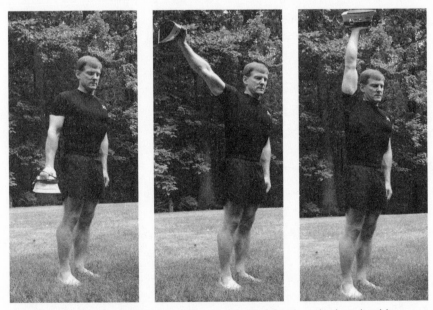

LATERAL EXTENSION. Lateral extension for trapezius, deltoid, and other shoulder muscles. This is another exercise that can be easily done with the room iron.

With a little imagination, you can use the items in your hotel room to help you exercise. *Remember that none of them were designed for exercise, and you need first to check them for stability and safety.* Exercise is never more important than avoiding injury or damaging hotel property.

It is wonderful to have a nice fitness center and the option of an in-room workout, but there are many options for outdoor exercise when the weather is good and the surroundings are safe. Usually, the hotel staff can advise you about walking or running paths, bike rentals, local parks, and outdoor exercise areas.

With a little imagination, you can use the items in your hotel room to help you exercise.

One of the great things about venturing outdoors to exercise is that it provides the opportunity to explore. Running in a new town is a great way to get oriented and discover new places and things. The sights, sounds, and smells can't be appreciated adequately from your hotel room or a fitness center. Passing though a market area or docks early in the morning can be exciting and memorable. Such sightseeing tours make the time and effort of your morning workout go by more quickly because you will be distracted by new experiences en route.

SUMMARY

Travel provides lots of opportunities to experience new foods. Remain conscientious about taking in fewer effective calories. *When the food's not right, take only a tiny bite.* Then move onto something else. . . but feel free to pack it up for home, where you can savor it over the next few days or share it with someone else.

Hydration can be more challenging when you are traveling, but don't ignore its importance. Plane rides, in particular, are dehydrating, and you need to be sure that water is readily available.

Protein bars can provide a quick source of protein after a workout far from home. Exercise away from home can be done imaginatively without leaving your hotel room, and exercising out-of-doors can give you great exposure to the surrounding sights, when weather and other conditions permit.

If you head out to a restaurant, you can often find dietary refuge in chicken or turkey entrees. Chefs know that many people look to turkey as a low-fat, healthy option. This chapter's recipe is one such option that you can prepare when you've returned home. Chicken is a great source of protein with very low caloric concern.

Chicken Breast with Wild Mushrooms

Yield: 4 servings

Calories per serving: 100; Protein per serving: 18g

1 garlic clove, minced

1 cup leeks, diced

1 Tbsp cracked black peppercorns

¼ cup vegetable stock

1 tsp chopped thyme (½ tsp dried)

2 cups fresh wild mushrooms, sliced

4 boneless chicken breasts, 4 oz each

1 cup chicken stock

Combine the garlic, pepper, and thyme. Rub the chicken breasts with the mixture. Cover and refrigerate until needed.

To prepare the sauce, cook the leeks in a large saucepan, in ¼ cup of the vegetable stock, until tender. Add the mushrooms and cook until tender. Add the remaining stock as needed to prevent the mushrooms from burning. Add the chicken stock and simmer until heated thoroughly. Use immediately or cool and refrigerate until needed.

Dry-sauté the chicken breasts to the desired doneness. Remove the meat from the pan, cover with the sauce, and garnish with a pinch of thyme. The sauce consists of the leeks, mushrooms, vegetable stock, and chicken stock, for a total of about 4 cups. 1 serving is about 1 cup of mushroom sauce per chicken breast.

8

Nutritional Supplements, Dietary Considerations, and Food/Medication Interactions

EVALUATING THE MERITS OF NUTRITIONAL SUPPLEMENTS

Before you spend money on vitamins or other supplements, consider whether they will be beneficial to your health. One of the most common errors that people make is to take nutritional supplements for which little evidence is available as to their effectiveness.

To further confuse the issue, many of the companies that manufacture supplements also pay for research studies to prove their products are the best. Many manufacturers even set up their own centers or institutions—usually under a different name. A spokesperson for such a group can make a claim without any obvious relationship to the manufacturer, thus making it difficult to assess the validity of those claims.

Therefore, vitamins and other nutritional supplements are best purchased from a reputable retail store, rather than through a mail-order outlet—and only after consulting with your doctor or other healthcare professional, who can determine whether a specific supplement might be helpful.

VITAMINS

Many people who are interested in diet and exercise also consider adding vitamins and other supplements to their diet. Few nutritional supplements, including vitamins, show any benefit unless a real deficiency exists. In some circumstances, taking additional vitamins can actually be harmful.

Little data supports the current widespread use of vitamin supplements. At the very least, they should not cause harm. The strongest data on vitamins for older adults probably relates to three vitamins: A, B complex, and D. Vitamin A supplements possibly cause harm for some older adults, but a great deal of data shows that vitamin D is associated with a wide range of benefits, from bones to balance.

Simply put, supplements should be used to treat an existing deficiency or prevent one from developing. Before deciding to take a vitamin supplement, you should first determine whether you are at risk for a deficiency—or at risk for toxicity from taking too much of the supplement. Table 8.1 includes questions that you should always ask when considering vitamin supplementation.

Supplements should be used to treat an existing deficiency or prevent one from developing.

Your evaluation of potential risks and benefits should include the cost of the supplement, how it is taken, how the effects (positive or negative) can be measured, and whether it might be helpful in treating specific problems. You need to consider carefully the specific reasons why you might take a vitamin or other nutritional supplement. For example, a vitamin A supplement might be important for some younger people who have specific visual issues or who are susceptible to infection, but it might not be necessary or appropriate for older adults. Vitamin B complex might be used to help manage cognitive issues or cardiovascular health, and it might be appropriate for some older adults. Vitamin D might be recommended for its effects on bone health, but its nonskeletal effects might be as important, or more important, for older adults.

TABLE 8.1 QUESTIONS TO BE ANSWERED BEFORE TAKING VITAMIN SUPPLEMENTS

This is generally termed "BARS," for *Benefit/Need, Assessment, Risk*, and *Schedule*

BENEFIT/NEED:

Is there evidence that supplementation would be helpful?

What are the indications for supplementation if vitamin status is normal?

Is there a general need in the population being considered for the supplement (for example, is there evidence of widespread deficiency in seniors in long-term care)?

Is there evidence that supplementation is needed only in deficient individuals?

ASSESSMENT:

How is deficiency measured?

Are follow-up measures needed?

RISK:

Is there evidence that supplementation would be harmful?

What is the likelihood of developing toxicity?

SCHEDULE:

How often should supplements be taken?

How much supplementation is needed?

For how long should the supplement be taken?

Vitamin A

Vitamin A is fat-soluble and—once present in the body—it takes months to become depleted. The current Recommended Dietary Allowance (RDA) for vitamin A is 5,000 I.U., and food supplements typically contain this amount or more. There is little reason to believe that vitamin A deficiency is a problem in adults in the United States or

Excessive vitamin A is linked to a potential risk of reduced bone density and/or increased risk of fracture. Canada. Additionally, excessive vitamin A is linked to a potential risk of reduced bone density and/or increased risk of fracture.

An article in the *Journal of the American Medical Association* (JAMA) showed an increased risk of mortality and morbidity with excess vitamin A and β-carotene. For these reasons, you should avoid vitamin A supplements, unless you have been told you are at risk of a real deficiency.

Vitamin B Complex

Vitamin B complex includes vitamins B_1, B_2, B_3, and B_6 (thiamine, riboflavin, niacin, and pyridoxine), as well as vitamin B_{12} and folate. Vitamin B_{12} and folate have been studied for their effects on cardiovascular and cognitive function, and there is some evidence that supplementation might be associated with an improvement in bone health and possibly a reduction in fractures. Although more research is needed to confirm this relationship, what has been done to date is intriguing because it applies to older adults who might be at risk for bone loss and fracture.

Optimal oral folic acid and vitamin B_{12} (cyanocobalamin) supplementation in older people who have deficiencies appears to be 1 mg per day, about 200 times the recommended daily intake. Supplementation with B_{12} and folate daily can be justified on a large scale in some settings, such as nursing homes, where deficits are common, benefits are likely, and the risk for adverse effects on health is small.

Vitamin D

Vitamin D deficiency is relatively common. It appears to be a problem for more than three-quarters of people over 70 and more than half of middle-aged adults, depending on the season and latitude. This makes vitamin D one of the most important vitamin supplements.

Traditionally, vitamin D has been associated with bone problems. Vitamin D deficiency is defined as a low levels of 25-hydroxyvitamin D (the molecule measured in a blood sample to assess vitamin D status) accompanied by either biochemical or physiologic abnormalities. Low vitamin D levels can result in bone loss, an increased risk for fracture, abnormal balance, and reduced strength. It is also associated with an increased risk of falls, impaired physical function, pain, and seasonal affective disorder (SAD). Giving vitamin D to people who are deficient addresses this problem. It also appears to be helpful in combating tuberculosis and some cancers.

The best way to replace vitamin D has not yet been determined.

The best way to take vitamin D has not yet been determined. Because it is a fat-soluble vitamin, taking daily supplements is not the only option. If daily dosing is chosen, it should consist of at least 800 I.U. per day, with doses of 1,600–2,000 I.U. per day for older individuals who are deprived of exposure to sunlight. Another option is to use less frequent megadoses of 50,000 I.U. of vitamin D_3 (cholecalciferol). Taking two such tablets once monthly is probably the easiest and cheapest way to take vitamin D. At the time of this writing, such a formulation was available without a prescription (www.bio-tech-pharm.com/catalog.aspx?cat_id=2).

Consult your physician or other healthcare professional before taking vitamin D more frequently, because of the serious possibility that vitamin D toxicity can lead to the development of markedly elevated calcium levels (hypercalcemia), which can have serious health consequences.

Vitamin D supplements can be recommended for many older adults, especially people who receive limited exposure to sunlight, such as those living in a long-term care setting. Some clinicians check vitamin D status with blood work no matter how oral vitamin D_3 supplementation is given (between 1,000–2,000 I.U. daily, or 50,000 I.U.–100,000 I.U. monthly). This blood work is not necessary routinely, but it might be recommended whenever a clinical concern arises about a person's vitamin D status—whether low or high.

OTHER SUPPLEMENTS

Vitamins are not the only supplements you might consider taking. For example, many older adults do not get adequate amounts of calcium, which is a mineral. The National Osteoporosis Foundation recommends 1,200 mg of calcium for people over 70 years of age, and for all postmenopausal women.

Protein supplements are also commonly used by older individuals.

Some examples of the many commonly used supplements are shown in Table 8.2. Note the amount of vitamin A in each, and keep in mind the concerns about vitamin A discussed earlier in this chapter. Many other supplements promise to help you gain weight, lose weight, build muscle, and burn fat, for example. Just remember, there is no magic pill for weight gain or loss. You need to be patient with respect to changes in weight and muscle mass, especially as you get older.

Two pounds a week is as much as you should expect to lose, although you might lose *slightly* greater amounts, depending on your level of exercise and how many effective calories you consume. No one should expect to safely lose more than half a pound a day for any length of time.

Use supplements *only* to provide what you can't get in your regular diet. For example, consider a supplement if you find it difficult to eat adequate amounts of protein. Most contain whey protein, a good source. Pay attention to what else is in a protein supplement. It should contain more than 15 grams of protein, with only small amounts of simple sug-

Consider a supplement if you find it difficult to eat adequate amounts of protein.

ars and overall calories, and only minimal amounts of other ingredients. *Always* read the labels. The packaging can often be deceptive, and you want to get the proper type and amounts of fats, vitamins, and total calories, in addition to protein. This applies to any supplement.

Any protein supplement, whether a bar or liquid (including powders to which you add milk or water), should meet the following requirement, with minimal extraneous ingredients:

TABLE 8.2 EXAMPLES OF THE VITAMIN CONTENT IN SOME SUPPLEMENTS (8 OZ)

Supplement	Boost®	Ensure®	Osmolite®
Vitamin A (IU)			
RDA 5,000 I.U.	1,250	1,250	625
Vitamin B			
Folate (mcg)	140	50	100
RDA 200 mcg	2.1	0.5	1.5
B_{12} (mcg)	0.7	0.5	0.5
RDA 2 mcg	5	5	5
B_6 (mg)	0.43	0.43	0.43
RDA 2 mg	0.38	0.38	0.38
Niacin (mg)			
RDA 20 mg			
Riboflavin (mg)			
RDA 1.8 mg			
Thiamine (mg)			
RDA 1.5 mg			
Vitamin D (IU)			
RDA 400 I.U.	150	100	50

- ▶ More than 15 grams of protein
- ▶ Less than 200 calories
- ▶ Less than 5 grams of simple sugar
- ▶ No trans-fats
- ▶ Reasonably good taste

DIET, EXERCISE, AND MEDICAL ISSUES

Some diseases that can't be cured *can* be altered by appropriate diet and exercise. Occasionally, they can become less severe or progress more

Some diseases that can't be cured can be altered by appropriate diet and exercise. slowly when modified by weight loss or the improved conditioning that comes with exercise. The effects of exercise include pain reduction and improvements in strength, balance, and walking ability.

Let's look at two diseases, common in older adults, that might be influenced by diet and exercise as discussed in this book, and that are especially good examples of what you can accomplish by following these principles.

Diabetes

Diabetes is very common among older adults, especially in those who are overweight. The term "diet-controlled" diabetes refers to people who maintain normal glucose levels as long as their weight remains in check through diet and exercise. For many diabetics, adherence to a diet low in simple sugars is also beneficial. Combining this with the principle of eating food with the right amount of effective calories will result in better control of glucose levels. Better sugar control might mean fewer medical problems in the long term.

Kidney Disease

Exercise and weight control can help manage kidney disease by reducing the likelihood of developing hypertension and atherosclerosis, which can impair renal function. Some experts encourage people with kidney disease to eat a low-protein diet. But, remember, losing weight without eating adequate amounts of protein might result in muscle breakdown. Although it is important to eat sufficient protein when maintaining a good exercise regimen, it is not necessary to exceed 100 grams of protein daily. Many older adults—with or without kidney problems—get inadequate amounts of protein. If you have kidney disease, you need to discuss any dietary regimen you're considering with your physician.

If you experience renal failure, your doctor will probably recommend that you take 0.25 mcg of 1,25 dihydroxyvitamin D (also called calcitriol or Rocaltrol®) at least 3–4 times a week, because of a problem in metabolizing vitamin D. This would be in addition to standard vitamin D supplementation.

Lactose Intolerance

Lactose intolerance is more common as we grow older, and it is often accompanied by nausea, bloating, and even diarrhea or vomiting. Lactose intolerance is caused by the lack of an enzyme called *lactase,* which is needed to break down *lactose*—a sugar found in milk—into a useable form. If you are eating extra dairy products in order to get more calcium, vitamin D, and protein, you need to deal with these symptoms when they first occur.

Treatment involves either avoiding lactose or taking a product such as Lactaid Fast Act®, which contains the necessary enzyme. Milk from cows does not contain lactase in any appreciable quantity.

Lactose is also present in many breads, cereals, and sauces. When you eat out, you can specify that you do not eat food containing dairy products, or simply take a lactase supplement before the meal.

After Surgery or Illness

Most acute illnesses, and surgery in particular, increase your body's energy and protein requirements. As a result, you can increase the amount you eat without increasing your weight. These energy requirements can be half again as much as your usual caloric needs for weight maintenance. Depending on the underlying disease, and/or the nature of the surgery, other nutritional needs might need to be addressed. A nutritionist can be very helpful in determining any increased nutritional requirements. Your physician can recommend a consultation with a nutritional specialist.

SORBITOL

Sorbitol is worthy of a brief mention. Occasionally, people who have been diagnosed with irritable bowel syndrome improve after lactose intolerance is detected and they are treated appropriately, and/or after counseling about avoiding sorbitol. Sorbitol is commonly used as a cathartic to induce a bowel movement; it is commonly found in sugar-free products, from candy to snowball cones.

Many people who change their diets in an attempt to lose weight switch to sugar-free products, resulting in symptoms such as bloating, abdominal discomfort, or diarrhea. In reality, these symptoms are related to the consumption of sorbitol.

DIET AND DRUGS

We do not recommend "diet pills" for older adults, because too many problems and adverse consequences are related to their use. Rather, this section deals with foods that can interfere with some prescription medications.

Some foods interfere with the absorption and action of many different types of medications.

Some foods interfere with the absorption and action of many different types of medications. For example, grapefruit can affect the absorption and metabolism of many drugs. Some drugs become ineffective when taken with any food at all. Table 8.3 lists some major food and drug interactions that you should avoid.

TABLE 8.3 FOOD AND DRUG INTERACTIONS

Drug(s)	Food(s)	Comment
Theophylline (used to treat some respiratory diseases)	High fat	Increase theophylline absorption
	High carbohydrate	Decrease theophylline absorption
Warfarin (Coumadin®) (commonly referred to as "blood thinners," these drugs are used to prevent the formation of blood clots and—as a result—strokes and heart attacks)	Foods high in vitamin K (e.g., broccoli, spinach, kale, turnip greens, cauliflower, and Brussels sprouts)	Decreases drug efficacy and promotes blood clotting
	≥400 I.U. vitamin E	May prolong bleeding times
Quinolones (antibiotics) such as ciprofloxacin (Cipro®), levofloxacin (Levaquin®), ofloxacin (Floxin®), trovafloxacin (Trovan®), tetracycline and other similar antibiotics (Achromycin®, Sumycin®)	Calcium-containing products such as milk, yogurt, vitamins or minerals containing iron, and antacids	Significantly decrease drug concentration
	Dairy products, antacids, and vitamins containing iron	Interferes with absorption and efficacy
Antifungals such as fluconazole (Diflucan®), griseofulvin (Grifulvin®), ketoconazole (Nizoral®), itraconazole (Sporanox®)	Dairy products (milk, cheeses, yogurt, ice cream), or antacids	Interferes with absorption and efficacy

(continued on next page)

TABLE 8.3 FOOD AND DRUG INTERACTIONS (CONTINUED)

Drug(s)	Food(s)	Comment
Monoamine oxidase (MAO) inhibitors such as phenelzine (Nardil®) or tranylcypromine (Parnate®), used as antidepressants and anti-anxiety medications	Processed, cheddar, blue, brie, mozzarella and Parmesan cheese; yogurt, sour cream; beef or chicken liver; cured meats such as sausage and salami; game meat; caviar; dried fish; avocados, bananas, yeast extracts, raisins, sauerkraut, soy sauce, miso soup; broad (fava) beans, ginseng, caffeine-containing products (colas, chocolate, coffee, and tea)	Severe headache and a potentially fatal increase in blood pressure (hypertensive crisis)
Medications affecting blood pressure, such as amiodarone (Cordarone®), astemizole (Hismanal®), atorvastatin (Lipitor®), budesonide (Entocort®),	Grapefruit (juice, segments, extract and certain related citrus fruits e.g., Seville oranges, pummelos, and	Alters absorption and efficacy

TABLE 8.3 FOOD AND DRUG INTERACTIONS (CONTINUED)

Drug(s)	Food(s)	Comment
buspirone (BuSpar®), cerivastatin (Baycol®), cilostazol (Pletal®), colchicine, eletriptan (Relpax®), etoposide (VePesid®), halofantrine (Halfan®), lovastatin (Mevacor®), mifepristone (Mifeprex®), pimozide (Orap®), quinidine (Quinaglute®, Quinidex®), sildenafil (Viagra®), simvastatin (Zocor®), sirolimus (Rapamune®), terfenadine (Seldane®), ziprasidone (Geodon®)	some exotic orange varieties)	
Bisphosphonates (for osteoporosis) such as alendronate (Fosamax®), ibandronate (Boniva®), risedronate (Actonel®)	Any food within 30-60 minutes	Blocks absorption
Digoxin (Lanoxin®) for some heart problems	Oatmeal	Fiber can interfere with absorption

Exercise and Disease

Many people equate a good diet with good health, but exercise can claim as much, or more, benefit because it promotes longevity. At least as important is the fact that "functional survival"—the ability to take care of yourself—is longer in people who exercise regularly.

Exercise has also been shown to relieve pain and painful syndromes such as *intermittent claudication,* which causes pain in the legs with prolonged walking. Studies have shown exercise-associated improvements in medical problems such as type 2 diabetes, cardiovascular diseases, osteoarthritis, and osteoporosis, as well as a reduced risk of developing a long list of other diseases.

Exercising in accordance with the principles and guidelines in this book promises a return that goes well beyond looking and feeling better.

Summary

A good diet balanced with exercise and careful supplementation offers a great opportunity to improve well-being as we grow older. Many people do not get adequate amounts of vitamin D. Knowing that certain diseases and medical conditions are more common in older adults, attention to foods that might interfere with medications can improve well-being. All the while, striving to stay active might be the best medicine of all.

Striving to stay active might be the best medicine of all.

The following recipe is a good example of a healthy and tasty dish that is relatively high in vitamin D and protein. It also contains omega-3 fatty acids and is an excellent option if you're concerned about cholesterol.

Seared Salmon with a Moroccan Spice Crust

Yield: 4 servings

Calories per serving: 175; Protein per serving: 15 g

1 lb salmon fillet

2 tsp cardamom seeds

2 tsp curry powder

2 tsp anise seeds

2 tsp coriander seeds

2 tsp black peppercorns

2 tsp cumin seeds

2 tsp caraway seeds

4 cups frisée, or any other hearty greens

Cut the salmon into four portions. Refrigerate until needed.

Combine the curry powder, cumin, caraway, cardamom, anise seeds, and black peppercorns. Grind coarsely in a spice grinder or coffee grinder.*

Rub each salmon portion with a generous amount of the spices. Dry-sear on both sides in a preheated sauté pan until browned and cooked to the desired doneness. If necessary, finish in a 350°F oven to prevent overbrowning.

Garnish plate with the frisée or other greens.

*Extra spice mix will keep for 4–6 weeks; store airtight in a dry, cold place.

9

Let's Be Specific: Defining What's Right for You

WHAT ARE YOUR NEEDS?

Everyone is unique. Depending on your age, weight, and—to some extent—your body type, you'll have different protein requirements, and you'll vary in how many calories you can consume and still lose weight.

A person who weighs 100 pounds might be able to maintain that weight with roughly 1,300 calories per day. For this person, weight loss requires reducing calories to about 1,000 a day, with about 40 grams of protein required.

A person weighing 150 pounds requires about 2,000 calories to maintain that weight, and a decrease to 1,500 calories might be needed to lose weight. About 60 grams of protein a day are required at this weight.

If you weight 200 pounds, eating 2,600 calories each day will produce little change in weight. A reduction to 2,000 calories a day is a good target for losing weight, and your protein requirements would be about 80 grams each day.

These figures are all somewhat dependent on having a lean body mass, or "body composition," with a high amount of muscle compared to fat. The greater the amount of muscle relative to fat, the greater the resting metabolic rate and the more energy that is expended at rest. Also, the more you exercise, the greater the weight loss you can achieve, because your base metabolism requires more calories over the course of the day. As we discussed in earlier chapters, exercise has an effect throughout the day, and exercise early in the morning can produce the most benefit. This also has an impact on protein requirements, which increase with greater amounts of exercise.

EXERCISES AND CALORIE EXPENDITURES

Your current body size affects the number of calories you will need for a given activity, as well as the type and duration of exercise that you do. For example, a 150-pound person doing aerobics for 15 minutes will burn about 100 calories. This same activity for someone who weighs 200 pounds will burn 135 calories. At 100 pounds, you can expect to use about 70 calories for this same exercise.

Brisk walking for 15 minutes will use about 50 calories if you weigh 100 pounds, 75 calories if you weigh 150 pounds, and 100 calories if you weigh 200 pounds. Golfing without using a cart for 3 hours will use about 500 calories if you weigh 100 pounds, about 800 calories if you weigh 150 pounds, and over 1,000 calories if you weigh 200 pounds.

Table 9.1 gives additional examples of exercises and associated calorie expenditures. These are rough estimates; other factors will affect how many calories you can actually use when performing a specific exercise. It is not necessary to be exact, nor should you walk around with a calorie calculator for your food intake and exercise expenditures. Rather, have a sense of the rough *effective calorie* content of the food you eat, and keep a general idea of the total calories you consume over a day. You should also keep in mind a general sense of the caloric benefit of your exercise routine.

As we have emphasized throughout this book, *effective calories* differ from the *absolute number of calories* in food. Some examples will

TABLE 9.1 CALORIES USED FOR SOME COMMON EXERCISES

Exercise	Weight (lbs)	Time (min)	Calories Burned
Aerobics	150	30	203
	200		270
	250		338
Bicycling	150	30	221
	200		294
	250		368
Bowling	150	30	108
	200		144
	250		180
Dusting	150	30	80
	200		106
	250		133
Gardening	150	30	162
	200		216
	250		270
Golf	150	180	783
	200		1,044
	250		1,305
Hiking	150	30	207
	200		276
	250		345
Housecleaning	150	30	122
	200		162
	250		203
Jogging	150	30	248
	200		330
	250		413
Doing Laundry or Making the Bed	150	30	72
	200		95
	250		120

(continued on next page)

TABLE 9.1 CALORIES USED FOR SOME COMMON EXERCISES

Exercise	Weight (lbs)	Time (min)	Calories Burned
Shoveling	150	30	203
	200		270
	250		338
Swimming	150	30	302
	200		402
	250		503
Vacuuming	150	30	85
	200		112
	250		141
Walking Dog	150	30	149
	200		198
	250		248
Brisk Walking	150	30	198
	200		264
	250		330
Washing Car	150	30	153
	200		204
	250		255
Weight Lifting	150	30	234
	200		312
	250		390

help to illustrate this concept. For most vegetables that grow above the ground, the amount of effective calories is about 85 percent of the absolute caloric carbohydrate content. Cereals and dairy products can be expected to register 90 percent or less than their total caloric content in effective calories. Processed bread has relatively little caloric expenditure before becoming available in the body and must be eaten sparingly if you are trying to lose weight. Most fruits and nuts will yield 85 percent or less in effective calories.

SUMMARY

Weight loss results from expending more calories than you eat. Formal and informal exercise (including basic chores around the house such as vacuuming or washing the car) can have a major impact on weight loss. Identifying foods that are lower in effective calories can make adjustments in your diet enjoyable and effective.

The next chapter considers a variety of food options designed to help you determine how to make the best selections you can to optimize weight control, based on the principles outlined in this book. Keeping effective calories in mind, and also being aware of energy expenditures, can result in excellent results without any real sacrifice.

The next recipe provides calories per serving and also a ballpark calculation of the calories you will use in preparing it—although it does not take into account activities such as shopping and carrying the groceries home. This should make the meal even more enjoyable!

Linguine with Asparagus, Fire-Roasted Tomatoes, and Olives

Yield: 4 Servings

Calories per serving: 196; Protein per serving: 14 g

Approximate calories in preparation: 60 per 20 minutes

1 Tbsp olive oil

2 tsp garlic, minced

¼ cup prosciutto, diced small*

1 lb green asparagus, thin, cut into 2-inch pieces

½ can (14.5-oz cans) fire-roasted tomatoes, diced**

½ cup spring onions, finely sliced

½ cup pitted kalamata olives, sliced

½ cup Parmesan, grated

8 oz spaghettini, dry

Heat 1 Tbsp olive oil in a large skillet. Add the garlic and sauté until aromatic, about 1–2 minutes. Add prosciutto and sauté for 1–2 more minutes.

Add the asparagus and tomatoes; cook until asparagus is tender, about 5–6 minutes. Add the olives and spring onions.

Cook the spaghettini according to the package directions until tender to the bite (al dente). Drain. Toss with all the vegetables.

Sprinkle with grated parmesan.

* Prosciutto can be replaced with any ham or Italian sausage.

** Fire-roasted tomatoes, available in cans, add a smoky, Southwestern touch to this dish.

10

A Final Review and Summary

EFFECTIVE CALORIES IN FOODS

So far, we've gone through the principles behind effective calories, and you should be comfortable with the merits of proteins compared to simple sugars when trying to shed pounds. It is worth giving some specific examples to help clarify.

Given the choice between sherbet and ice cream, many people would look at the total number of calories and choose the scoop of sherbet. However, the calories in the sherbet mostly consist of simple sugars, while the ice cream includes protein and fat, as well as carbohydrates. There are about 135 calories in 100 grams of sherbet, compared to 200 calories in 100 grams of ice cream. Because of the energy needed to metabolize the protein and fat into usable energy forms, however, the discrepancy between the two is actually much closer in terms of effective calories.

Similar logic comes into play when comparing 100 grams of almonds or 100 grams of M&M's®. The almonds have slightly more calories (598) than the candy (513), but because the calories in the candy mostly consist of simple sugars the *effective calories* of the nuts is comparable to or better than the candy. Other nutritional benefits, such as protein and calcium, make the almonds the healthiest choice.

The principles throughout the text can be further illustrated with this example: At lunch, you may be offered a selection from a sandwich tray. Given the choice between your basic ham (2 slices or 2 oz) and cheese (1 slice or 1 oz) sandwich with mustard on whole wheat bread, or a tuna fish salad sandwich on a bagel, you should choose the ham and cheese sandwich (about 350 calories) and pass on the tuna salad on a bagel (over 800 calories).

While fruits are generally felt to be healthy, fruit juices may not be the best choice when trying to lose a few pounds. For example, given the option between a glass of orange juice or skim milk at breakfast, the juice might not be the better choice. Skim milk has about 80 calories, while orange juice has about 100. The main contribution to calories in the milk comes from protein and simple sugars, while almost all of the calories in the orange juice come from simple sugars. Thus, skim milk is the preferred product for weight loss. If you like orange juice, however, you can choose "light" options that have about half the calories as regular juice. These may be fortified with calcium and vitamin D, in amounts comparable to that in milk, making this an excellent choice with fewer calories, even when effective calories are taken into account.

Although effective calories are important, some foods with high concentrations of simple sugars may sometimes be the better choice. For example, a half-grapefruit has 32 calories versus 80 calories for an omelet, assuming that a no-fat, nonstick spray is used for cooking. The grapefruit is essentially all simple sugars, while the omelet is loaded with nutrients, including protein. The taste factor might make the decision for you. If you're really in the mood for grapefruit, go for it. In reality, both are so low in effective calories, especially if you use egg substitutes, that you could have both.

FOOD AND MEDICATIONS

Some foods interfere with medications. The earlier list in Chapter 8 should be helpful, but always ask your pharmacist, physician, or nurse about food interactions with newly prescribed medications. For example, if you were considering the breakfast selection mentioned above while taking the cholesterol-lowering drug Atorvastatin® and the allergy medicine Terfenadine®, you should definitely choose the omelet. Knowing that the grapefruit interferes with both of these medications will outweigh the caloric basis for your decision.

YOU DON'T NEED TO BELONG TO A GYM TO EXERCISE AND LOSE WEIGHT

The preceding chapters should make it clear that many ways to exercise don't require elaborate facilities. Some activities that we don't even think of as exercise are excellent calorie burners.

Consider two scenarios. You decide to stay home and do some chores. You vacuum, do a load of laundry, make the beds, dust, spend half an hour gardening, then do another half hour of general house-cleaning. Your friend decides that she "needs to get into shape" and foregoes a similar routine at home in favor of going to an aerobics class 15 minutes away by car and a half hour hike at a trail she likes that is a 30-minute drive from her home. On the way home from her hike, she stops to reward herself with a soft ice cream cone. You celebrate as well with a single scoop of ice cream. Who made out better?

In addition to getting your house in shape, you won from a caloric perspective as well. Your total energy expenditure would be over 500 calories, while your friend's would be about 400. Your choice of a single scoop of regular ice cream provides 150 calories, giving you a net loss of 350 calories. Your friend's choice of a soft ice cream cone is close to 250 calories, giving her a net loss of 150 calories. Over the same period of time, you made out far better calorie-wise (and you saved on gasoline).

TEN TIPS FOR GETTING INTO GOOD SHAPE AND STAYING THERE

▶ *Limit your effective calories.* This means minimizing your intake of simple sugars and keeping effective calorie counts per day to a level that allows weight loss or maintenance of a desired weight. Intake of foods with trans-fats should also be limited.

▶ *Exercise in the morning whenever you can.* Early daily exercise increases your metabolism throughout the day, giving you a calorie-burning dividend for that early rise investment!

▶ *Drink ample amounts of water.* Even mild dehydration causes fatigue and slows metabolism by 3 percent. This means you're burning fewer calories. Especially in older adults, thirst might be misinterpreted as hunger. Consuming fluids often decreases hunger, and it contributes to physical expansion of the stomach, which also helps to quell hunger.

▶ *Eat some form of protein within 30 minutes of exercising.* Protein is a building block for muscle. This will help to assure that the calories being burned come from fat and not from muscle.

▶ *Avoid eating after 8 P.M.* A slower metabolism after sleeping can contribute to fat deposition, so avoid the after-dinner snacks later in the evening.

▶ *Walking and household chores are great exercise.* You don't always have to go to a gym to exercise (see Table 9.1).

▶ *You don't need to eat three meals a day.* The total *effective calories* you eat each day will affect your weight. You can choose to have small meals throughout the day, or satisfy yourself with two meals and a snack. Recommended daily amounts of nutrients are based on averages, and many nutrients store very well. Many people choose to fast on certain days for spiritual or other reasons. As long as other days bring sufficient nutrients, an occasional fast day is fine. Also, an occasional splurge (but no more than once a week) is okay.

▶ *Only a few supplements, such as vitamin D and calcium, can be generally recommended, even for older adults.* Taking a multiple vitamin with minerals might be helpful if your diet is not sufficient but—for most people—other supplements are not recommended unless you have specific nutritional deficiencies.

▶ *Exercise with good form at a controlled pace after a relaxed warm-up.* Any type of jerking motion or traumatic exercising technique increases the likelihood of injury. As we get older, recovery from injury takes longer. For an 80-year-old person, after 5 days of bed rest, it can take almost a month of exercise to get back to the level of functional capacity present before the period of bed rest.

▶ *Following an exercise routine with a friend will increase your chances of staying with your program.* Knowing that someone is counting on you can provide even more motivation to show up. Additionally, socializing with friends also helps promote health and longevity.

The next chapter provides a great variety of recipes from one of the world's most creative chefs. They incorporate the principles discussed throughout the book and are absolutely delicious. With a little planning and preparation, you'll look better, feel better, live better, and, most importantly, be healthier.

11

Reveling in Recipes: Chef Speckamp's "Calorically Kind" Culinary Delights

In this chapter, Master Chef Rudy Speckamp provides some recipes that reflect the philosophy of *Fit At Fifty and Beyond*. They are savory and relatively simple, although a few are included that might require a little more effort for a really special occasion. These recipes are sure to pleasantly surprise your guests when they learn how healthy each serving is—should you choose to reveal that bit of information! They are low in simple sugars, very reasonable in terms of general calories, and particularly good for you because of their reduced effective calories due to the balance of protein, fat, and complex carbohydrate. The recipes avoid trans-unsaturated fatty acids (trans-fats), and generally use monounsaturated or polyunsaturated fats when needed. The number of calories and the amount of protein per serving are listed for each recipe.

Don't worry too much about tracking every calorie or gram of protein. Eat with a general sense of each. Your goal is to consume adequate amounts of protein each day, with 10–20 grams eaten within about half an hour of your daily workout. Chapter 9 gives detailed information on calorie and protein intake that you can use as a guide. Based on that information, you can determine which meals and how many servings will best allow you to meet your health and weight goals.

We intentionally chose not to list other nutrients—or even fat and carbohydrate content. Most of the carbohydrates will be complex, and by now you should understand that fats are only avoided because of their overall calorie content or type. As a result, you don't need to know more about fats beyond the overall caloric content of each serving.

Finally, this is not intended to be a cookbook! These recipes are meant to be fun to prepare, enjoyable to eat, and in keeping with the principles in the book. Some will be great for special occasions. Chef Speckamp has kept the reader in mind with ingredients and instructions that everyone should be able to find and follow. As you'll find, healthy eating can also be delicious eating.

Bon appétit!

To Start: Soups, Chowder, & Chili

Soups are a great choice for dinner. Whether light or hearty, they can be prepared ahead of time, frozen, and taken from the freezer and served after a busy day.

Chilled Gazpacho

Yield: 2 quarts

Calories per 1 cup serving: 105; Protein per serving: 3 g

1 quart chicken or vegetable stock

2 Tbsp extra-virgin olive oil

2½ cups tomatoes, peeled, seeded, and diced

1 Tbsp balsamic vinegar

1 cup green pepper, diced

1 Tbsp chopped tarragon

¾ cup scallions, split, diced

2 tsp Worcestershire sauce

½ cup cucumber, peeled, seeded, diced

1 tsp lime juice

½ cup celery, diced

½ tsp salt

1 jalapeño chili, seeded, diced

½ tsp Tabasco sauce

3 Tbsp chopped basil

¼ tsp ground white pepper

Crouton Garnish

1 garlic clove

2 slices bread cut into cubes*

2 tsp extra-virgin olive oil

Combine all the ingredients and purée until smooth. Chill for 8 to 12 hours, to allow the flavor to develop.

To make the garnish, sauté the garlic clove in olive oil until aromatic. Remove the garlic and add the bread cubes. Sauté until crisp and lightly browned.

Garnish each serving of soup with a small amount of the croutons.

* Prepackaged croutons can be substituted if desired.

Manhattan Clam Chowder

Yield: 2 quarts

Calories per 1 cup serving: 163; Protein per serving: 18 g

This chowder requires about 45 minutes preparation and about 45 minutes for cooking. It can be cooked in advance, refrigerated, and frozen in serving-sized portions. Reheating will develop the flavor and makes for a quick meal during the week.

2 dozen cherrystone clams, shucked, juice reserved; canned or frozen can be substituted

3 plum tomatoes, peeled, seeded and chopped

2 bacon slices, minced

1 cup tomato juice

½ cup onion, diced

2 potatoes, peeled and diced

½ cup carrot, medium dice

1 sprig fresh thyme, or ½ tsp dried

½ cup celery stalks, medium dice

½ cup sliced leeks, medium dice

1 sprig fresh marjoram, or ½ tsp dried

½ cup fennel, medium dice

½ cup bell pepper (red or green) seeded and diced

1 bay leaf

7–8 cracked black peppercorns

4 garlic cloves, minced

½ tsp salt or to taste

4 cups clam broth

Chop the clams into large pieces. Cook the bacon in a soup pot over medium heat until it is crisp, about 5 minutes.

Add the onion, carrot, celery, leeks, fennel, pepper, and garlic; stir to coat evenly with the bacon fat. Cover the pot and cook over low heat until the onion is translucent, 6 to 8 minutes. Add the clam broth, reserved juices, tomatoes, tomato juice and bring to a simmer.

Add the potatoes, thyme, marjoram, bay leaf, and peppercorns. Simmer over low heat for 15 to 20 minutes, or until the potatoes are tender.

Add the clams and simmer for 5 minutes more or until the clams are tender and cooked just until their edges have curled slightly; do not overcook or the clams with toughen.

Adjust the seasonings and serve.

Vegetarian Bean Chili

Yield: 2 quarts
Calories per 1 cup serving: 270; Protein per serving: 10 g

This is another recipe you can prepare ahead of time, freeze in serving-sized portions, and serve later.

1 lb dried black beans
2 Tbsp cumin seeds, toasted, ground
¼ cup olive oil
2 cups onion, diced
1 Tbsp coriander seeds, toasted, ground
1 Tbsp minced garlic
1 cup celery, diced
1 Tbsp hot paprika
1 cup red pepper, diced
6 cups tomatoes, peeled, seeded, and diced
1 cup green pepper, diced
½ oz cilantro, chopped
1 jalapeno chili, minced
1 tsp salt
½ tsp crushed black peppercorns

Soak the beans for 4 hours in enough water to cover by 3 inches. Drain and rinse with cold water.

Combine the beans with enough fresh water to cover in a large stockpot. Simmer until the beans are tender, about 1½ hours, adding more water as necessary to keep the beans covered. Drain the beans and reserve until needed.

Heat the oil in a large soup pot. Add the onions and sauté until the onions are caramelized.

Add the garlic and sauté for 1 minute. Add the celery and sauté for 1 minute. Add the peppers and spices. Sauté until aromatic, about 3 minutes.

Add the tomatoes and beans. Simmer until the vegetables are tender and the flavors have developed, about 20 minutes.

Just before serving, season the chili by adding the cilantro, salt, and pepper.

Chilled Potato-Basil Soup

Yield: 1½ quarts

Calories per 1 cup serving: 80; Protein per serving: 2 g

With half & half—Calories per 1 cup serving: 160; Protein per serving: 4 g

With half & half (fat-free)—Calories per 1 cup serving: 93; Protein per serving: 3 g

1 bacon slice, chopped

¼ tsp freshly ground black pepper, or to taste

1 yellow onion, chopped

2 Idaho potatoes, peeled and sliced

Tabasco sauce to taste

4 cups chicken broth

1 plum tomato, finely diced

1 bay leaf

2 Tbsp shredded fresh basil (If using dried, cut amount in half)

½ cup half & half (optional)

½ tsp salt or to taste

Cook the bacon in a soup pot over medium heat until crisp, about 5 minutes.

Add the onions and sauté, stirring frequently, until they are tender and translucent, 6 to 8 minutes.

Add the potatoes, broth, and bay leaf, and simmer until the potatoes are tender enough to pierce easily with a fork. Remove and discard bay leaf.

Let the soup cool slightly and then puree it in a blender or food processor until smooth.

Transfer the soup to a bowl; cool to room temperature and refrigerate overnight.

If necessary, the consistency may be adjusted by adding additional broth or water. Add half & half to the chilled soup if desired. Taste for seasoning and add salt, pepper, and Tabasco sauce as desired. Top with diced tomato and basil just before serving.

Pumpkin and Coconut Soup
(Gaeng Lieng Fak Thong)

Yield: 1½ quarts

With Coconut milk—Calories per 1 cup serving: 427; Protein per serving: 9 g

With Coconut cream—Calories per 1 cup serving: 587; Protein per serving:
   11 g

If you have access to an Asian market, you'll be able to find lemongrass, tamarind, and fish sauce; they are also available in supermarkets in some areas.

2 lbs pumpkin (canned may be used)

½ cups tamarind, chopped (optional)

¼ cup fresh lime juice

1 quart clam juice or chicken stock

4 shallots or red onions, chopped

½ cup fish sauce (nuoc nam) if using clam juice

1 stalk lemongrass, chopped

1 tsp chilies

1 bunch basil

1 quart coconut milk or cream

If using fresh pumpkin, peel and seed.

Dice, place in a bowl, and sprinkle with lime juice. Leave to stand while preparing other ingredients.

Mix shallots, chilies, and lemon grass in food processor and blend to a fine paste.

Pour contents of food processor and coconut milk into a large saucepan. Stir until dissolved. Bring to boil. Add tamarind, clam juice or chicken sauce, and simmer for 10 minutes. Then add pumpkin pieces and cook until tender.

Add additional stock or water as needed.

Season with fish sauce. Return mixture to food processor and blend to puree. Serve garnished with coconut milk/cream and basil leaves.

Entrees: Seafood

Grilled Yellowfin Tuna with (Optional) Citrus Salad

Yield: 4 servings

Calories per serving 364; Protein per serving: 29 g

1 lb trimmed yellowfin tuna fillet

Ground black pepper to taste

½ tsp salt

½ cup red onions, very thinly slice

½ lemon, zest only

½ tsp black pepper

½ lime, zest only

¼ cup peanut or macadamia oil

½ tsp cornstarch

¼ cup vegetable stock

1 cup pink grapefruit sections, cut into bite-sized pieces

¼ cup orange juice

1 oz roasted jalapeños

1 cup white grapefruit sections, cut into bite-sized pieces

1 cup shaved fennel bulb

1 cup orange sections

¼ cup blood orange sections

¼ tsp salt

Cut the tuna into ten 3 ½-oz portions. Refrigerate until needed.

Julienne the lemon and lime zest. Place the zest in a small saucepan, cover with cold water, and bring to a boil. Drain and repeat the blanching process twice, beginning with cold water each time. Reserve the zest until needed.

Combine the cornstarch with enough vegetable stock to form a thin liquid. Bring the remaining stock to a boil in a small saucepan and add the liquid. Stir until the stock thickens. Remove from the heat and cool to room temperature.

Combine the thickened stock with the orange juice, jalapeno, salt, and pepper. Slowly whisk in the oil. Reserve the dressing until needed.

Combine the citrus sections. Reserve until needed.

Season the tuna with a pinch of salt and pepper and place on an oiled grill. Grill to the desired doneness.

While the tuna is grilling, heat 4 oz of the citrus sections with 1 Tbsp of the dressing and a pinch of the lemon-lime zest in a sauté pan just until warmed.

Place some of the shaved fennel in the center of a heated plate. Top the fennel with red onion, and place the citrus salad above the fennel. Slice the tuna and fan below the fennel. Drizzle the plate with 1 Tbsp of the vinaigrette and serve immediately.

Marinated Fish with Herbed Tomatoes and Lentil Bulgur Salad

Yield: 6 servings

Calories per serving 210; Protein per serving: 32 g

With Salad & Tomatoes—Calories per serving 455; Protein per serving: 49 g

For a quick mid-week dinner, eliminate the lentil bulgur salad and substitute a salad of your choice.

6 5–oz portions sturgeon or any firm fish such as swordfish or monkfish

3 cloves garlic, minced

2 Tbsp teriyaki light marinade

1 tsp ginger, minced

⅓ cup fish stock or bouillon

Salad (Optional)

1 cup bulgur wheat, cooked

1 cup green lentils, cooked

½ red bell pepper, cleaned, seeded, diced

½ green pepper, seeded, diced

½ yellow pepper, cleaned, seeded, diced

¼ cup white onion, finely diced

1 tsp cumin

2 Tbsp cilantro, chopped

1 lemon, juice only

2 Tbsp rice vinegar

1 Tbsp olive oil

Salt and cracked pepper to taste

Tomatoes

6 plum tomatoes, cored, washed, cleaned, sliced lengthwise

1 Tbsp fresh herbs, snipped

Preheat oven to 375°F. Rub fish with garlic, teriyaki, and ginger. Marinate for 30 minutes. In a hot pan, sear on all sides until evenly browned. Finish cooking in oven until done. Skim any drippings from pan. Add stock. Stir constantly and reduce volume by one-third. Remove drippings from pan and allow to cool. Set aside to mix with salad.

Remove fish from oven. Slice into 1–1½" thick steaks. Serve on top of lentil bulgur salad.

For salad, combine bulgur wheat with lentils in mixing bowl. Add peppers, and toss. Add onion, cumin, cilantro, lemon juice, vinegar, and olive oil. Adjust seasoning with pepper and a little salt. Add cooled pan drippings, combine thoroughly. Allow flavors to develop for approximately 30 minutes. Just before serving, taste and adjust seasoning.

For tomatoes, preheat oven to 200°F. Toss plum tomatoes with fresh herbs then place on baking rack. Roast gently for 2 hours.

Roasted Fish with Balsamic Vinegar and Shallots

Yield: 4 servings

Calories per serving 188; Protein per serving: 32 g

2 tsp olive oil

⅓ cup balsamic vinegar

1½ lbs monkfish or halibut fillet, in one piece

1 Tbsp honey

4 medium shallots, thinly sliced

½ cup fresh Italian (flat-leaf) parsley leaves, for garnish

½ tsp coarsely ground black pepper

Preheat the oven to 425°F.

In a heavy, medium skillet, bring the oil to the smoking point over high heat. (The oil must be very hot or the fish will stick.) Add the fillet and brown it quickly on both sides, about 1½ minutes total.

Put the fillet into an oiled roasting pan and roast until it is softly resilient to the touch, about 9 minutes. Remove the fillet to a warmed platter.

Add the shallots, pepper, vinegar, and honey to the roasting pan. Place the pan over low heat and deglaze it, stirring and simmering until the shallots have softened, 3 to 4 minutes.

Slice the fillet into 1-inch pieces. Pour the sauce on top and garnish with the parsley. Serve immediately.

Salmon Fillet with Smoked Salmon and Horseradish Crust

Yield: 4 servings

Calories per serving 416; Protein per serving: 40 g

4 salmon fillets, cut into four 6-ounce portions
¼ cup lime juice
2 tsp shallots, minced
2 tsp garlic, minced
2 tsp black peppercorns, crushed

Crumb Mixture
2 tsp shallots, minced
1 tsp garlic, minced
⅜ cup butter
1½ cups bread crumbs, fresh

2 Tbsp horseradish, prepared

Preheat the oven to 350°F.

Rub the salmon fillets with the lime juice, shallots, garlic, and peppercorns.

To prepare the crumb mixture, sauté shallots and garlic in the butter until they are aromatic, about 1 minute.

Combine the sautéed shallots and garlic, the bread crumbs, smoked salmon, and horseradish in a food processor and process to a fine consistency.

Place salmon fillets on baking pan. Cover each fillet with a few spoonfuls of the crumb mixture. Bake in a 350°F oven until salmon is opaque pink on the outside and just beginning to flake, 6–7 minutes.

Entrees: Meats

Turkey with Tomato-Basil Sauce

Yield: 4 servings

Calories per serving 251; Protein per serving: 31g

This recipe is ideal for preparation ahead of time, freezing that portion you won't serve immediately for a quick mid-week meal. It's also ideal for a buffet.

1 lb boneless, skinless turkey breast

Tomato-Basil Sauce

1 oz tomato paste

1 cup chicken stock

2 Tbsp onion, chopped

8 black peppercorns

2 Tbsp carrot, chopped

4 thyme sprigs

2 Tbsp celery, chopped

1 bay leaf

¼ cup dry white wine

8 parsley stems

Dry Spice Mix

3 Tbsp salt

1 Tbsp dried oregano

3 Tbsp dry mustard

1 Tbsp ground coriander

1 Tbsp coarse-ground black pepper

1 Tbsp ground celery seed

1 Tbsp dried thyme

1 Tbsp peanut oil

¾ cup all-purpose flour

1 cup tomatoes, peeled, seeded, and diced

2 Tbsp basil cut into thin strips (1 Tbsp dried)

Slice the turkey breast into 8 2-oz portions. Refrigerate until needed.

To make the sauce, roast the tomato paste, onion, carrots, and celery in a 375°F oven until browned. Add the wine and transfer the mixture to a large stockpot. Add the stock, peppercorns, thyme, bay leaves, and parsley. Simmer for 2 hours. Strain the sauce through a fine-meshed sieve and return to the heat. Simmer for 45 minutes or until a sauce consistency is achieved. Keep warm.

Combine the ingredients for the spice mix.

Heat oil in a sauté pan. Dredge turkey slices in the spice mix and then in the flour. Sauté until golden brown on both sides.

Filet Mignon with Wild Mushrooms

Yield: 4 servings

Calories per serving 365; Protein per serving: 42g

This is a good recipe for a party because the sauce can be made ahead of time.

4 5–oz portions filet mignon

2 fl oz Madeira wine

½ cup leeks, julienne-cut

1 tsp chopped thyme (½ tsp dried)

½ cup chicken stock

1 tsp chopped sage (½ tsp dried)

¾ lbs fresh wild mushroom, sliced

½ tsp crushed black peppercorns

Cook the leeks in the stock until tender. Drain and reserve.

To make the sauce, heat the stock in a saucepan. Add the mushrooms and allow them to cook briefly. Add the wine, thyme, sage, and pepper. Simmer and reduce to a sauce consistency. Add the leeks. Use immediately or cool properly and refrigerate until needed.

For each serving: Dry-sauté each filet mignon to the desired doneness. Remove the meat from the pan and add ¼ cup of the sauce. Serve the filet on a pool of the sauce.

Lemon Chicken with Toasted Pearl Couscous

Yield: 4 Servings

Calories per serving 780; Protein per serving: 82g

Note that these are very large servings and could easily be cut in half.

Lemon Glaze

4 oz chicken stock

4 oz lemon juice

2 Tbsp lemon zest

2 Tbsp honey

½ tsp ginger, chopped

½ tsp star anise, ground

½ tsp ground black pepper

2 whole cooked rotisserie chickens

Toasted Pearl Couscous

2 cups pearl couscous*, toasted, cooked

Chicken stock as needed

2 Tbsp basil, cut into strips

1 Tbsp tarragon, chopped

1 Tbsp black olives, chopped

To prepare the chicken glaze, combine the chicken stock, lemon juice and zest, honey, ginger, star anise, and black pepper in a blender and process until smooth.

Transfer the processed mixture to a saucepan, bring to a boil, and cook until reduced by half. If necessary, thicken with corn starch to achieve a glaze-like consistency.

Generously brush the glaze onto the hot chicken before serving. Divide each whole chicken into two halves, then slice each half into three pieces.

In a non-stick skillet, reheat the pearl couscous with a little chicken stock, then add the basil, tarragon, and black olives.

Place the couscous in the center of the plate, and arrange the chicken slices on top.

* The grains of pearl couscous (also called Israeli couscous) are much larger than those of regular couscous. Regular couscous or orzo are acceptable substitutes.

Entrees: Vegetarian

Farmer's Salad

Yield: 4 Servings

Calories per serving 370; Protein per serving: 15g

4 cups frisée or other hearty lettuce

8 bacon, sliced

16 asparagus spears, blanched

3 yellow beets, roasted, peeled and sliced

1 tsp shallots, minced

½ tsp garlic, minced

1 tsp Dijon mustard

¼ cup white balsamic vinegar

¼ cup hazelnut oil

4 eggs, hard-boiled, cut in halves

½ cup sourdough bread, cut into cubes

½ tsp salt

½ tsp ground black pepper

In a sauté pan, cook the bacon to render the fat. When the bacon is crisp, let drain on a paper towel and reserve.

To prepare the vinaigrette, combine the shallots, garlic, mustard, balsamic vinegar, and hazelnut oil in a bowl and whisk until combined. Set aside.

Just before serving, toss the frisée, asparagus, sliced yellow beets in the vinaigrette until evenly coated. Adjust seasoning with salt and pepper, if necessary.

Arrange the frisée, asparagus, sliced beets, and hard boiled eggs on a dinner plate. Top with crisp bacon slices and croutons.

Penne al'Aglio

Yield: 4 Servings

Calories per serving 330; Protein per serving: 14g

1 Tbsp olive oil

1 Tbsp garlic, minced

1 tsp red crushed pepper

1 (14.5 oz) can fire-roasted tomatoes

½ cup parmesan, grated

½ cup basil, cut into thin strips

½ (16 oz) box penne pasta

Heat olive oil in a medium sauce pot. Add the garlic and red pepper. Sauté until garlic becomes aromatic, about 1–2 minutes. Add the tomatoes and let simmer until liquid is reduced by half, about 15–20 minutes.

Cook pasta according to the package directions. Drain. Toss with tomato sauce. Sprinkle with cut basil and grated parmesan.

Wild Mushroom Casserole

Yield: 4 Servings

Calories per serving 76; Protein per serving: 4.5g

1 Tbsp olive oil

2 garlic cloves, minced

½ pound shiitake mushrooms, quartered*

½ pound cêpes mushrooms, quartered

½ pound chanterelle mushrooms, whole

2 rosemary sprigs

2 thyme sprigs

¼ tsp salt

½ tsp ground black pepper

Heat the olive oil in a large sauté pan; add the garlic and shallots and sauté until translucent.

Add the mushrooms and herb sprigs and cook, stirring frequently, until the liquid is reduced and the mushrooms are just moist.

Remove the sprigs of rosemary and thyme and adjust the seasoning with salt and pepper.

* Any mushroom medley will work, although the flavor will vary slightly.

Veggie Burger

Yield: 4 servings

Calories per serving 452; Protein per serving: 27g

Without Cheese—Calories per serving 325; Protein per serving: 17g

½ cup rolled oats, toasted (not instant)

¼ cup pecans, coarsely chopped

1 Tbsp olive oil or canola oil

½ cup green onions, chopped (including green tops)

2 tsp garlic cloves, minced

1½ cups mushrooms sliced

½ cup cooked rice

⅓ cup white cheddar cheese, grated

⅔ cup tofu, firm, mashed

½ cup Egg Beaters®

3 Tbsp parsley, chopped

½ cup dry bread crumbs

¼ tsp salt

Garnish

6 mozzarella slices, fresh

1 cup salsa, preferably fresh

Heat the oil in a sauté pan. Over moderate heat, sauté the onions, garlic, and mushrooms until softened and lightly colored. Add the oats and continue to cook for another 2 minutes, stirring constantly. Turn off the heat and cool mixture. When cool, turn onto a cutting board and use a knife to chop the mixture.

Combine the chopped onion-mushroom mixture with the rice, cheese, tofu, Egg Beaters®, parsley, bread crumbs, and almonds and stir to combine. Season to taste with salt and pepper. Shape into 12 small patties, approximately ¾-inch thick and 2 inches wide. Sauté or broil until golden and crisp on the outside.

Top with a slice of fresh mozzarella and a teaspoon or two of salsa. Serve immediately.

VEGETABLES

Sautéed Spinach

Yield: 4 Servings

Calories per serving 80; Protein per serving: 7g

2 tsp extra virgin olive oil

1 tsp garlic, minced

4 oz shallots, julienne

2 pounds spinach leaves, rinsed and drained

Salt and pepper, to taste

Heat the oil in a large sauté pan; add the garlic and shallots and sauté until translucent.

Add the spinach leaves, along with any water still clinging to them. If the leaves are very dry, add a few teaspoons of water or stock to the pan.

Cover tightly and steam for a few minutes until the leaves are barely wilted. Uncover and reduce any excess liquid.

Season with salt and pepper. Toss and serve while hot.

Pan-Steamed Lemon Asparagus

Yield: 4 Portions

Calories per serving 74; Protein per serving: 1g

2 bunches asparagus

2 Tbsp olive oil

¼ cup shallots, minced

4 tsp garlic, minced

¼ cup lemon juice

¼ cup white wine

Trim the bottoms off the asparagus spears so that they are equal in length.

Heat the oil in a large sauté pan over medium heat. Cook the shallots and garlic until translucent, about 2 minutes. Add the asparagus and cook for 4 to 5 minutes.

Add the lemon juice and white wine to the pan. Cover and steam the asparagus until cooked through, about 3 minutes. Serve immediately.

Sautéed Broccoli Rabe

Yield: 4 Portions

Calories per serving 86; Protein per serving: 6g

2 pounds broccoli rabe, or regular broccoli

1 Tbsp olive oil

1 tsp garlic, chopped

1 tsp shallots, chopped

½ tsp salt

½ tsp ground black pepper

⅛ tsp red pepper flakes

Wash the broccoli and remove any tough stems and very large leaves.

Blanch in a saucepot with boiling salted water for 2 to 3 minutes. Drain and cover with cold water to stop the cooking process.

Heat the olive oil in a large sauté pan. Cook the garlic and shallots until translucent.

Add the broccoli and cook until heated through. Season with salt, ground black pepper, and red pepper flakes.

Broccolini with Orange-Sesame Sauce

Yield: 4 Servings

Calories per serving 116; Protein per serving: 7g

2 pounds broccolini or broccoli

Orange-Sesame Sauce

1 cup orange juice

2 Tbsp honey

1 Tbsp ginger, peeled and grated

1 Tbsp lemon juice

2 tsp sesame oil

2 tsp sesame seeds

Salt and pepper to taste

Blanch the broccolini in a saucepot with boiling salt water until just tender, about 6 to 8 minutes.

To prepare the sauce, combine the orange juice, honey, and ginger in a small saucepan and bring to a boil.

Cook until the sauce reduces and thickens, about 3 minutes.

Stir in the lemon juice and sesame oil and cook for an additional 2 minutes. Season with salt and pepper to taste.

Arrange the broccolini on a plate. Ladle enough sauce over the broccoli to form a light glaze. Sprinkle with sesame seeds and serve.

EGG DISHES/BRUNCH

Savory Turkey Quiche

Yield: 8 Servings

Calories per serving 320; Protein per serving: 30 g

With Low-fat Boursin—Calories per serving 242; Protein per serving: 12 g

1 Tbsp vegetable oil

½ cup red bell pepper, diced small

½ cup green bell pepper, diced small

½ cup potatoes, diced small

3 eggs

1 Tbsp cornstarch

2 cups evaporated skim milk

4 oz Boursin cheese

1 Tbsp fines herbs

Salt to taste

Ground white pepper to taste

Pinch ground nutmeg

8 oz turkey breast, cooked, diced small

8-inch pie shells, pre-baked (either your recipe or frozen)

Heat the vegetable oil in a skillet; add the red and green peppers, and sauté until they are tender. Remove from heat and let cool.

Blanch the diced potatoes in boiling salted water. Drain and let cool while preparing the custard.

To prepare the custard, whisk together the eggs, cornstarch, and evaporated skim milk. Mix in the Boursin cheese and fines herbs and season with salt, pepper, and nutmeg.

Spread the sautéed peppers, blanched potatoes, and diced turkey evenly into the pie shells. Top with the Boursin-custard mixture.

Bake in a 350°F oven until the center of the quiche is set, about 40 to 45 minutes.

Remove from the oven and allow to cool slightly. Serve with your favorite salad.

Spanish Potato Omelet

Yield: 8 Servings

Calories per serving (including Sofrito) 317; Protein per serving: 19g

¼ cup olive oil

2 cups Idaho potatoes, medium dice

10 oz sofrito, cooked (recipe follows)*

4 cups spinach leaves, washed

16 eggs

2 Tbsp cilantro, chopped

8 slices bacon, cooked until crisp, crumbled

In a large non-stick skillet, heat 2 Tbsp of the olive oil. Add the potatoes and cook over low heat until tender, stirring every 2 minutes to prevent sticking. Add the sofrito and spinach and cook until the spinach is wilted.

Remove from heat and let cool.

In a large bowl, whisk the eggs with the cilantro. Add the sofrito mixture and stir until combined.

Add 1 tsp of the remaining oil into a non-stick skillet and heat until it just begins to smoke. Add ¾ cup of the egg mixture to the pan; reduce the heat and cook without stirring until the eggs begin to set. When the eggs begin to lightly brown on the bottom, turn the omelet over and cook until the second side is golden brown.

Sofrito*

Yield: 10 ounces cooked sofrito

¼ cup onions, chopped

1 garlic clove, chopped

¼ cup green bell peppers, small dice

1 cup red bell peppers, diced small

1 cup tomatoes, seeded, chopped

½ tsp achiote paste*

⅛ tsp dried oregano

1 Tbsp cilantro, chopped

¼ tsp salt

1 pinch ground black pepper

Combine all ingredients in a saucepan and cook over low heat until the mixture is soft.

* Achiote paste is generally available in Hispanic stores—you could substitute with red chili paste.

Frittata Toscana

Yield: 4 Servings

Calories per serving 462; Protein per serving: 38g

1 Tbsp olive oil

1 cup Vidalia onions, diced

1 cup green bell peppers, small dice

1½ cups Yukon Gold potatoes, diced and cooked

½ cup prosciutto, diced

½ bunch green onions, cut on the bias

1 cup tomatoes, seeded and diced

8 eggs

Salt to taste

Ground white pepper to taste

½ bunch basil, sliced into thin strips

½ cup fontina cheese, grated

½ cup parmesan cheese, grated

Heat the olive oil in a skillet; add the onions and green peppers, and sauté for 2 to 3 minutes. Add the potatoes and continue to sauté until they are tender, about 10 minutes. Add the prosciutto, green onions, and tomatoes and continue to cook until heated through.

In a mixing bowl, beat the eggs and season with salt and pepper. Stir in the basil, grated fontina cheese, and parmesan cheese.

Pour the egg mixture over the vegetable–meat mixture.

Reduce the heat to low, cover the skillet, and cook until the eggs are nearly set, about 4 to 5 minutes.

Remove the cover and place the skillet under a broiler to lightly brown the edges.

Remove from heat and cool slightly, then cut into wedges. Serve with your favorite salad.

Resources

WEB SITES

http://www.lightenupamerica.org provides information about healthy eating and physical activities.

http://www.caloriesperhour.com/ is a good source for determining the nutritional content of foods and the number of calories burned with exercise and various activities.

http://www.nia.nih.gov/HealthInformation/Publications/Exercise Guide/ has great tips on exercise for older adults from the National Institute on Aging.

http://www.bio-tech-pharm.com/catalog.aspx?cat_id=2 is a good source for vitamin D_3 (cholecalciferol) without a prescription.

http://www.eatright.org/cps/rde/xchg/ada/hs.xsl/nutrition.html gives consumer-oriented resources from the American Dietetic Association.

http://www.seniorhealthcare.org/ gives senior-focused information on fitness and nutrition in its "hot health topics" section and includes an "ask-the-expert" section.

http://www.nia.nih.gov/HealthInformation/Publications/healthy eating.htm gives sound advice for seniors on eating right.

BOOKS

Living SMART: Five Essential Skills to Change Your Health Habits Forever by Joshua C. Klapow and Sheri D. Pruitt; DiaMedica Publishing: New York, 2007.

Successful Aging by John Wallis Rowe, M.D., and Robert L. Kahn; Dell Publishing, a Division of Random House, Inc: New York, 1998.

The Mayo Clinic Plan for Healthy Aging by Edward T. Creagan (Editor-in-Chief); Mason Crest Publishers: Philadelphia, 2002.

DVDs

Tai Chi for Older Adults by Paul Lam; 60 minutes; produced by East Acton Video, 1998.

Tai Chi Exercises for Seniors by Bob Klein; 60 minutes; produced by Tapeworm Inc., 2000.

COOKBOOKS

The Good Housekeeping Cookbook: 1,039 Recipes from America's Favorite Test Kitchen by The Editors of *Good Housekeeping*; Hearst Corporation: New York, 2007.

365: No Repeats–A Year of Deliciously Different Dinners (A 30-Minute Meal Cookbook) by Rachael Ray; Clarkson Potter/Crown Publishing Group/Random House: New York, 2005.

The New Betty Crocker's 30-Minute Meals for Diabetes by The Betty Crocker Editors; Clarkson Potter/Crown Publishing Group/Random House: New York, 2008.

The New American Heart Association Cookbook, 7th Edition by the American Heart Association; Clarkson Potter/Crown Publishing Group/Random House: New York, 2007.

American Heart Association Low-Salt Cookbook, 3rd Edition: A Complete Guide to Reducing Sodium and Fat in Your Diet by the American Heart Association; Clarkson Potter/Crown Publishing Group/Random House: New York, 2007.

The Martha Stewart Living Cookbook: The New Classics by Martha Stewart Living Magazine; Clarkson Potter/Crown Publishing Group/Random House: New York, 2007.

The Fannie Farmer Cookbook: Anniversary by Marion Cunningham and Lauren Jarrett; Knopf Publishing/Random House: New York, 1996.

Emeril's Delmonico: A Restaurant with a Past by Emeril Lagasse; William Morrow Cookbooks/Harper Collins: New York, 2005.

Eat This Book: Cooking with Global Flavors by Tyler Florence; Clarkson Potter/Crown Publishing Group/Random House: New York, 2005.

Home Cookin' with Dave's Mom by Dorothy Letterman; Atria Books/Simon & Schuster: New York, 1996.

Weight Watchers New Complete Cookbook 3rd Edition by Weight Watchers; Wiley: Hoboken, N.Y., 2007.

The New Moosewood Cookbook (Mollie Katzan's Classic Cooking) by Mollie Katzan; Ten Speed Press: Berkeley, CA, 2000.

O, The Oprah Magazine Cookbook by the Editors of *O Magazine*; Hyperion/HarperCollins: New York, 2008.

500 Low-Carb Recipes: 500 Recipes from Snacks to Dessert That the Whole Family Will Love by Dana Carpenter; Fair Winds Press/Quayside Publishing Group: Beverly, MA, 2002.

The Gourmet Cookbook: More than 1000 Recipes by John Willoughby, Zanne Early Stewart, and Ruth Reichl, Editor; Houghton Mifflin: Boston, MA, 2006.

The Joy of Cooking: 75th Anniversary Edition by Irma S. Rombauer, Marion Rombauer Becker, and Ethan Becker; Scribner/Simon & Schuster: New York, 2006.

How to Cook Everything: Simple Recipes for Great Food by Mark Bittman; Wiley: Hoboken, N.Y., 2006.

The Whole Foods Allergy Cookbook: Two Hundred Gourmet & Homestyle Recipes for the Food Allergic Family by Cybele Pascal; Vital Health Publishing: Ridgefield, CT, 2005.

Better Homes and Gardens New Cookbook: 11th Edition by Better Homes and Gardens Editors; Bantam Books/Random House: New York, 1997.

The Sugar Solution Cookbook: More Than 200 Delicious Recipes to Balance Your Blood Sugar Naturally by The Editors of *Prevention* and Ann Fittante; Rodale Books: Emmaus, PA, 2006.

Index

Note: Boldface numbers indicate illustrations; italic *t* indicates a table.